Visualising Health Care Practice Improvement

Innovation from within

RICK IEDEMA
PhD, USyd
Research Professor and Director
Centre for Health Communication, University of Technology
Sydney

JESSICA MESMAN
PhD, UM (Univ Maastricht)
Department of Science and Technology Studies
Maastricht University

and

KATHERINE CARROLL
PhD, UTS
Australian Research Council Postdoctoral Research Fellow
Centre for Health Communication, University of Technology
Sydney

With contributions from
Chris Ball, Gordon Caldwell, Cor Kalkman, Corine Kooyman,
Twan Mulder, Elizabeth van Rensen and Bas de Vries

Radcliffe Publishi
London • New York

Radcliffe Publishing Ltd
33–41 Dallington Street
London
EC1V 0BB
United Kingdom

www.radcliffehealth.com

———————————————————————

British Library Cataloguing in Publication Data

A catalogue record for this book is available from the British Library.

ISBN-13: 978 184619 450 4

The paper used for the text pages of this book
is FSC® certified. FSC (The Forest Stewardship
Council®) is an international network to promote
responsible management of the world's forests.

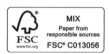

Typeset by Darkriver Design, Auckland, New Zealand
Printed and bound by TJI Digital, Padstow, Cornwall, UK

Visualising Health Care Practice Improvement
Erratum

FIGURE 2.1 The quality broom
Reproduced from Lillrank P, Liukko M. Standard, routine and non-routine processes in health care. *Int J Health Care Qual Assur*. 2004; **17**(1): 39-46 with permission from Emerald.

FIGURE 2.2 Direct and indirect pathways from communication to health outcomes
Reproduced from Street RL Jr, Makoul G, Arora N, *et al*. How does communication heal? Pathways linking clinician- patient communication to health outcomes. *Patient Educ Couns*. 2009; **74**(3): 295–301 with permission from Elsevier.

Vignette 3.1 Video stills reproduced from Iedema R. Creating safety by strengthening clinicians' capacity for reflexivity. *BMJ Qual Saf*. 2011; **20**(Suppl. 1): S83-6 with permission from the BMJ Publishing Group Ltd.

FIGURE 5.3 Researcher introducing main focuses to the video-reflexive focus group
Reproduced with permission from SAGE. First published in Carroll K, Iedema R, Kerridge R. Reshaping ICU ward round practices using video-reflexive ethnography. 2008. *Qual Health Res*. 2008; **18**(3): 380-90.

Contents

Contents

Preface

THIS BOOK'S POINT OF DEPARTURE IS THE FOLLOWING QUESTION: why is it that in spite of all the health policy reforms, clinical practice innovations, increasing intersectoral interdependencies and new medical and information technologies, so little has changed in the way we research and evaluate health care? Don't these changes cry out for new ways of being studied and appraised? And don't our approaches to clinical practice innovation cry out for being reinvented too? Surely, we cannot continue to wheel out research and evaluation paradigms, improvement approaches and methods that were designed for twentieth-century problems and twentieth-century health care, and assume they will be able to make sense of the problems we experience and the care we provide in the twenty-first century?

This book's response to this question is that these changes necessitate a new paradigm of health service research, evaluation and improvement. Such new paradigm adopts approaches and methods that embrace complexity. These approaches and methods can account for the vicissitudes of front-line care, the activities of front-line staff and the experiences of patients and families. Indeed, the point of departure for these approaches and methods is where care happens: they take their cue from how care happens in the 'here and now', and they orient their attention to how those involved provide and experience that care.

Our interest in hospital-organisational change and health reform started with Pieter Degeling's thesis that health care should pay attention to 'the work'. The Work. For Pieter, The Work is that which is done from moment to moment in the name of health care provision. The continuing blind spot in health reform, in his view, is that its statistical, economic and process management arguments rarely include consideration of how The Work is performed, organised and communicated.

One way in which The Work comes into view for clinicians is when they become patients. As patients, they apprehend care as the behaviours and communication enacted by the clinicians around them. Another way in which The Work is foregrounded is when we listen to narratives or watch footage of patients telling stories about their care or clinicians providing care. The reason The Work comes into view for patients is because they are there, all of the time. Seen from this perspective, The Work unfolds in ways that are often at odds with how clinicians understand it and experience it.

Until recently, the people in charge of running health services and policy reform initiatives – mostly clinicians – have tended to regard The Work as a given, as uninteresting, dismissing it as too obvious, and classifying its complexities as 'unimportant noise'. More important are the numbers we generate about numbers of beds, patient throughputs, delays in discharge processes, surgery cancellations and unplanned readmissions. Numbers dominate the approaches we deploy to tackle health care problems. Numbers *as such* are taken to be neutral, impartial and objective. Numbers are *the* currency for trading knowledge and grounding decisions.

However, now things are changing. Recent developments provide evidence of The Work as it unfolds in the here and now rapidly becoming considered as critical to understanding health care processes and outcomes. We witness a growing interest in patients' experiences, their views on outcomes and their participation in decision-making (Johnson and Abraham, 2012). There are initiatives such as 'experience-based co-design', which involves patients and clinicians sharing experiences and using these to redesign processes and spaces (Bate and Robert, 2007). Another recent development is the rise in popularity of 'rounding'. Rounding involves clinicians regularly catching up during the day with colleagues and patients to discuss issues and problems that arise as the day goes on (Studer, 2003). The power and effect of these developments lies in their capacity to personalise care, its processes and its outcomes.

The here and now is also being brought into focus through the roll-out of sophisticated computer systems deploying 'statistical process control'. Statistical process control provides increasingly fine-grained representations of what goes on in a service from moment to moment (Hart and Hart, 2002). Such systems can show how many patients there are in a ward at midday today, when these patients are expected to be discharged, what time of day their discharge is expected to happen, what bottlenecks exist where, and so forth. These systems' principal mode of representation remains statistical and numerical. In contrast to patients' narratives and staff rounding, therefore, these systems operate at several removes from care as *in situ* activity. Their power and effect are not to personalise care, but to technicalise it.

A powerful way of personalising *and* technicalising the here and now is by videoing care processes as they happen. The resulting footage can be analysed, focusing on whether clinicians adhere to technical rules and clinical procedures (Mackenzie and Xiao, 2003; Michaelson and Levi, 1997). Equally, footage of *in situ* work may be used to foreground experience and its complexity. Rather than using such footage to gauge what is done against pre-existing rules and compare it with pre-existing standards, it may be used to initiate discussions with clinicians and patients, to hear how they make sense of the resulting footage, how they experience it and what they can do with it.

In our work we drew on years of video feedback research (Bottorff, 1994; Hargie and Morrow, 1986; Heath and Hindmarsh, 2002; Pink, 2007) to shape an approach that enables those who appear in the footage to work with it, comment on it. Intuitively, we felt that video offered such an immediate connection with the here and now. We wanted to see whether this approach might enable people to translate their use of such footage into a novel kind of sense-making, and whether that might produce new ways of experiencing and enacting *in situ* care. In showing the footage back to those in the footage, we essentially sought to produce 'reflexivity' – the ability on the part of those involved to experience, frame and enact *in situ* care 'from under a different aspect' (Wittgenstein, 1953).

In 2002 we got our first opportunity to study clinicians in video feedback on the back of a larger government-funded project on the computerisation of clinical test ordering. The promising outcomes of that study (Forsyth, 2006; Iedema *et al.*, 2007) led us to submit further grants targeting front-line practitioner involvement in videoing and viewing clinical workplace footage, redesigning their own work processes and reshaping relationships. Along the way, this video-feedback-change process came to be termed 'video-reflexive ethnography'. 'Reflexive', because we insisted on involving those whose work was captured in the footage, and saw them as central to producing outcomes from the project – changes in practice, in relationships, in understandings. This was not simply about reflection, but about internalising the ability to frame care 'from under a different aspect': reflexivity. 'Ethnography', because we wanted to capture and understand 'naturally occurring work processes'.

As we engaged in this work, our ethnographic focus soon shifted from being retrospective ('what is going on'), to being prospective ('what does this feedback make possible'). This is because we learned that trying to understand the here and now is like trying to fix ocean waves: what we are looking at is constantly moving, and the most we can take away with us is some general idea about what is happening and where things are going. That is, the image we end up with is not of a fixed object, but of a *potential*, a range of possibilities inherent in what is going on. The feedback process made us further realise that clinicians and patients are critical players in shaping (and reshaping) this potential – the wide variety of contextual 'forcing functions' (Norman, 1988) and systems constraints notwithstanding. No technology or system is ever without limitations and constraints (Berwick, 1996). Therefore, the aim to create the perfect, flawless system will never be realised. We will never be able to give up on training users of those systems in how to work within their limits, compensate for their shortcomings, accommodate their constraints and capitalise on their potential.

The achievements of our early projects were so persuasive that we now rarely study anything without using video. Video footage always throws an unexpected light on things – whether these things are team meetings and team communication, infection control practices, clinical handovers and ward rounds, end-of-life care or medical supervision. Video reveals what linguistic and numerical renderings of care practices can never show: the multilayered flow of work, its dynamics and complexities, and the deep interconnectedness of people, technologies and spaces. This is what fascinates people: they come to apprehend activity and themselves as actors 'from under a different aspect'. Upon viewing footage of their own work, people often exclaim, 'My god that's amazing, I've never seen myself do that!' – suggesting that people can perform activities without being fully aware of how or why they enact them. For us, this raised questions about intentionality and agency – aspects of human behaviour with which practice improvement initiatives rarely concern themselves (Russell *et al.*, 2008). Surely, if actors enact habits without conscious intent or awareness, what could they hope to achieve in response to a call for practice change? As Dewey stated almost a hundred years ago, changing practice in such a situation is like 'whistling for wind' (Dewey, 1922).

Then, in 2004, we received funding from the Australian Research Council for another video study, part of which was Katherine's doctoral study (Carroll, 2009). Inspired by the project's senior researcher, Debbi Long, and her ethnographic experience and inventiveness, this project produced many exciting outcomes (Iedema *et al.*, 2010; Iedema *et al.*, 2006). Then, in 2008, Katherine and Rick came across Jessica's work. Jessica had taken to heart the question about why not more incidents happen in health care, and she was applying her 'science and technology studies' focus to study neonatal intensive care in the Netherlands. When Jessica came out to Sydney for a couple of months and worked with us on a project to develop a video-based practice-improvement programme, we had much to talk about. What became apparent was that Jessica's approach to enabling practitioners to appreciate and recognise their own unique abilities and *in situ* accomplishments complemented our video-based approach to practice improvement and involving clinicians in considering the change potential embedded in their existing ways of working.

Our discussions led us to appreciate that everyday practice itself is rich with *affect*. Following Deleuze, affect is defined as the swirl of influences prefiguring what we are, say and do in the here and now (Deleuze, 2005). Video makes affect visible and tangible in that it captures the subtle interplay of people's movements, faces and gestures – a choreography of which we in ordinary life are only marginally or intermittently aware. Video puts the affective dimensions of social interaction into relief.

This is particularly true for those who view themselves on screen. Essentially, video implicates us as actors. We feel implicated in video footage because it confronts us with an entirely new perspective from which to apprehend who we are, what we say and what we do. This is not purely about knowing or 'seeing' – it is about experiencing. Its intense effect is due to the moving image's special qualities. It differs radically from the spoken phrase or the still photo, as Massumi explained in his book *Parables for the Virtual* (2002). The moving image transforms, he said, because it alters our perception and therefore our sense of existence. That is precisely what it does every time we train the camera on ordinary processes in care, and when we display the resulting footage to stakeholders in that care. Because it comes as a series of moving images, video unfolds the performance of care in all its dynamic complexity. It bares who we are and what we do in a way that is neither excessively confronting (as verbal feedback from a colleague might be), nor too forgiving (like, say, a flattering photo). This is because footage reveals that we are deeply connected to others and to ongoing events.

In doing so, footage (and watching footage of ourselves) places us within a new paradigm of thinking and experiencing. It highlights fluidities in what we do and say together. It reveals seamless continuities in how activities unfold. It highlights social and practical connectedness. All this points to the unacknowledged and powerful *logic* that is embedded in everyday activities but which we are generally led to take for granted. This logic explains why watching ourselves say and do things, while sometimes confronting, can be both intriguing and reassuring. Intriguing because video shows us entrained by the complex social processes that structure our interpersonal and professional lives. Reassuring because video reveals the high degree of *sociality* that is embedded in action. Put differently, video reveals the high degree of social and organisational *imbrication* that we ignore in order to continue to experience ourselves as 'rational, intentional individuals'.

Preface

Our imbrication in social activity is particularly evident in video footage because it foregrounds the habituated dimensions of our actions and decisions. As Bourdieu explained several years ago now, habitus is the set of habituations that defines us as social beings (Bourdieu, 1990). Habitus is our personal repertoire of ways of being, doing and saying. However, habitus is drawn from the social reservoir of available and possible ways of being, doing and saying. The aetiology of habitus reaches back into our childhood and social background. Its present manifestation is what we take as given in the form of our personhood. Its future is circumscribed by whether and to what extent we can secede from our childhood and from its typical manifestations and influences, to reinvent ourselves and our habitus (Sloterdijk, 2009).

Video aids such secession. It perturbs habitus by bringing everything closer to us on the screen, and by at the same time distancing us from what we (and those we identify with) do and say. Loosening our ties to habitus, video footage expands our activity repertoire. It grants us a view of the broader social reservoir of opportunities and possibilities, and of opportunities and possibilities that extend beyond that reservoir. This is not about giving up who we are; it is about expanding our repertoire of actions and identifications, extending our habitus.

This brings us to the second pillar of the present book: Jessica's work on *exnovation*. Exnovation captures two ideas. First, the idea that it is possible to observe the exquisite skills already present among practitioners (Idea 1). Later in the book we come to talk about this skill as 'phronesis', drawing on one of Aristotle's terms. Second, the idea that innovation should and can come from within, not without. Innovation from within (Idea 2) becomes possible when we become aware of the doings, sayings and beings in which we are embroiled and implicated (our habitus: our repertoire of habituations). Innovation from within becomes possible when we gain an outsider perspective on the dynamics, effectiveness and impact on us and others of these doings, beings and sayings. These doings, sayings and beings are the soil, if you will, from which new forms of activity and identity can and need to grow. Indeed, there is no other soil for changes and innovations from which to grow.

Framed thus, change is not principally about adopting solutions from elsewhere. Rather, change is conditional on people exploring whether proposed solutions suit existing habituations. Exnovation is the term we use for this process of exploration, discovery, secession and renewal. This makes clear, too, that change is in the first instance about exploring the soil from which innovations need to grow, more so than the innovations themselves. Unless we are clear about our existing relationships, activities and habituations, and unless we take the opportunity to think about what particular innovations may mean for those relationships, activities and habituations, innovations are likely to fall on fallow ground.

Moreover, given we are concerned in this book with social and organisational innovations, the point about exploring relevance and connection becomes even more critical. Here we are not principally concerned with adopting a new surgical instrument or a novel drug. Social and organisational innovations are more akin to changing how we conduct ourselves, hold our bodies, and the like. Also, changing ourselves and our conduct is a complex matter. To tell someone to straighten their shoulders may produce appropriate posture for a few seconds, or even minutes, but such posture is unlikely to last. Changing posture involves the demanding process of becoming attentive to how we hold ourselves, inhibiting our habituated ways of standing and walking, and through practice teaching ourselves to adopt and normalise a new way of holding ourselves. Here, as in social and organisational change, learning springs from an ongoing exploration of our own bodies in action, of their reaction to inhibiting what feels 'natural', and of their receptivity of new norms and conducts (Shusterman, 2008).

These are the main components and premises of this book. The reader can engage with our extended arguments in the first four chapters, or skip these and move straight to examples of video-based exnovation in action in the second part of the book (Chapters 5–8). In the book, we use the terms professional, practitioner and clinician interchangeably. We talk about researchers, but this term refers to anyone wanting to intervene in contemporary forms of clinical practice, and this may include junior clinicians doing projects, quality and safety officers, managers who appreciate that observing front-line practice is more profitable than sitting in endless meetings, or clinicians who are passionate about practice improvement. As you move through the book, you will meet several such clinicians, as we have invited them to share their stories using video in the pursuit of exnovation.

Rick Iedema
Jessica Mesman
Katherine Carroll
January 2013

Acknowledgements

We thank the Australian Research Council for its financial support (Discovery Grants DP0879002, DP0556438 and DP0450773 and Linkage Grant LP0347042). We also thank all the clinicians and patients who participated in the projects described here.

About the authors

Katherine Carroll PhD, UTS is an Australian Research Council Postdoctoral Research Fellow at the Centre for Health Communication, University of Technology, Sydney. Her current research uses video and ethnographic methods to understand how donor human milk is used in neonatal intensive care units in Australia and the United States.

Rick Iedema PhD, USyd is Research Professor and Director of the Centre for Health Communication at the University of Technology, Sydney. He is also Fellow of the Academy of Social Sciences of Australia and Associate Editor of the journal *Health Expectations*. Rick's research investigates the rising complexity of health service provision.

Jessica Mesman PhD holds a senior position at the Department of Science and Technology Studies at Maastricht University. Her book *Uncertainty in Medical Innovation: Experienced Pioneers in Neonatal Care* won the Sociology of Health and Illness Best Book of the Year 2009 Award. Jessica's research applies a science and technology studies approach to patient safety in, among others, intensive care and neonatology, and to decision-making processes in critical care medicine.

List of contributors

Chris Ball is employed at the New South Wales Agency for Clinical Innovation, Sydney, Australia, and he has a background in critical care nursing. He is a Visiting Fellow at the Centre for Health Communication, University of Technology, Sydney.

Gordon Caldwell is a consultant physician at Worthing Hospital, Brighton, and at Western Sussex Hospitals NHS Trust in the United Kingdom. His aims include improving quality, safety, effectiveness, efficiency and patient and staff satisfaction while retaining staff and cutting costs of overheads.

Cor Kalkman MD, PhD is an anaesthesiologist and Research Professor at the Division of Anesthesiology, Intensive Care and Emergency Medicine, University Medical Center Utrecht, the Netherlands.

Corine Kooyman is an infection control practitioner at the Maastricht University Medical Center, the Netherlands.

Twan Mulder is a paediatrician and neonatologist at the Maastricht University Medical Center, the Netherlands.

Elizabeth van Rensen MPH, PhD is a senior researcher Quality and Safety at the University Medical Center Utrecht, the Netherlands. She is a biomedical scientist and has a master's degree in public health.

Bas de Vries BSc is a trainer and senior consultant Quality and Safety at the School of Medical Sciences, University Medical Center Utrecht, the Netherlands. He has a nursing background and has worked as an educator for intensive care and emergency department medicine.

Glossary

Accountability – accountability refers to the imperative imposed on people to describe (offer an account about) what occurs to others.

Adaptive practice – adaptive practice refers to practice shaping itself or being shaped by actors to suit emerging circumstances. An individual's activities can be said to be adaptive when they reconfigure themselves or are reconfigured in a dynamic way to accommodate changing circumstances. For example, when faced with a medical emergency team call, an intensivist clinician may need to curtail and hand over intensive care unit tasks in favour of meeting the urgent call. Their task reconfiguration is likely to impact on the intensive care team. The success or failure of such task reconfiguration will depend on the degree to which colleagues are capable of adaptive practice. Enacting adaptive practice harbours evidence of team members sharing a degree of 'distributed intelligence'.

Affect – affect refers to a range of phenomena to do with feeling. One of these phenomena is people's capacity for action, and the increase in affect resulting from the expansion of one's capacity for action (Deleuze, 2005; Ticineto-Clough 2008). Critical to the discussion in this book is the notion that our capacity to act is enhanced by our 'power to be affected'. As Michael Hardt notes: 'The greater our power to be affected . . . the greater our power to act [because] every increase of the power to act and think corresponds to an increased power to be affected – the increased autonomy of the subject, in other words, always corresponds to its increased receptivity' (Hardt, 2007: x).

Clinician – the term clinician refers to any professional undertaking clinical tasks: doctors, nurses, and allied health professionals.

Collective competence – collective competence refers to what collectives of people can do thanks to belonging to the group (Boreham, 2004). Boreham's point is that collective competence exceeds the sum of individuals' knowledge and capability.

Complexity – complexity is a term used to describe states of affairs whose origins and ways of unfolding into the future are 'overdetermined'. Overdetermination points to such states of affairs being influenced by and incorporating diverse, intersecting, non-linear and generally unpredictable phenomena. The word complexity derives from the Latin word *complexus* which signifies 'entwined' and 'twisted together'. Complexity thus involves phenomena interacting in ways that are not fully predictable. Complexity is to be distinguished from both order, which is fully explainable with reference to a limited number of rules, and total disorder, a state of affairs that accommodates no rules at all. Finally, complexity can be said to increase when the variety and interdependency of parts or aspects of the state of affairs in question increase.

Consultant – a consultant is a senior, fully qualified specialist doctor.

Deficit thinking – this term refers to a deficiency perspective on (clinical) practice. Such perspective takes errors, failures and transgressions as central both to understanding that practice and to improving it.

Distributed intelligence – the concept distributed intelligence is cognate to Hutchins' 'distributed cognition' (Hutchins, 1995), but harbours an important difference. Distributed cognition closely resembles 'collective competence' in what it seeks to foreground; namely, the shared nature of social action and the connectedness that characterises actors' knowledge about what is done and why. For Hutchins, the critical and distinguishing aspect of collective action is that actors complement each other's knowledge and action, contributing different kinds of knowledge and action to the emerging practice as a whole. For us, distributed intelligence highlights, besides actors complementing each other's actions, actors reflecting on these dynamic processes and deducing principles from them for future activity. Thus, distributed intelligence points not merely to the speed but also the quality of feedback among practitioners. The more explicit and *meta-discursive* actors' feedback, the more actors are able to expand their potential for adaptive practice, and hence the more intelligent, and effective, the practice.

Ethnography – ethnography refers to a method developed and favoured by anthropologists for studying cultures and practices. The ethnographer spends time with the people they are trying to understand and describe. To achieve this, they observe events and practices and learn from 'informants'. The ultimate aim is to absorb and crystallise out the logics (the structures that underpin and that may characterise such people's ways of being, doing and saying) that govern how people mean and feel.

Exnovation – exnovation throws light on the details of *in situ* practice (De Wilde, 2000). Exnovation reveals and enhances what practitioners do to accomplish effective, continuous and safe patient treatment. Rendering these details explicit by visualising them and talking about them opens up the opportunity for practitioners to become aware of them. This, in turn, may transform the group's tacitly held collective competence into a more explicit and pro-active distributed intelligence. Exnovation does this by engendering a discourse about what happens ('this is happening now') and by eliciting meta-discourse about how practitioners work, talk and think together ('this normally happens, that could happen, and something else should happen').

Flexible systematisation – flexible systematisation is derived from Timmermans and Berg's (2003) discussion about flexible standardisation. The term flexible standardisation refers to the collaborative construction of *standards*. We suggest this concept is more productively interpreted to refer to the collaborative construction of *systems* of practice. Here, 'systems' encompass process designs, protocols and checklists, as well as practices that mobilise and thereby *realise* those resources. The phrase flexible systematisation emphasises that we are not concerned in the first instance with making practitioners meet standards and benchmarks, but with engendering practitioner awareness of and discussion about existing and potential systems of practice.

Futurising the present – this phrase refers to actors' constant assessment and forward projection of scenarios in which they are or may be embroiled, or by which they may be affected (Ticineto-Clough, 2008). Given the rising complexity of everyday organisational life, actors are increasingly called on to futurise the present to maximise their agency in practical situations and optimise the outcomes of their actions. Futurising the present becomes more possible when actors open themselves to and passively observe surrounding circumstances (*see* 'passivity competence' below).

Forcing functions (Norman, 1988) – forcing functions manifest as constraints on what people do, and they force people to act in particular, pre-planned ways. Forcing functions are embedded in language (guidelines, protocols), in technologies, and in spaces.

Habitus – habitus is originally an Aristotelian notion referring to the totality of predispositions that define a person and their conduct. Bourdieu (1990) emphasised the biographical, social–historical and memory dimensions of habitus. Habitus thus refers to the recurrent, predictable and patterned dimensions of personhood and persons' activity potential.

Hologrammatic – this term serves to highlight the multi-layered nature of something that might ordinarily seem single-layered (e.g. video footage). The layering referred to here is to do with interpretive potential: something is hologrammatic if and when it offers a variety of views on something. The term hologram refers to an object whose surface harbours multiple pictorial effects.

Intensivist – an intensivist is a clinician who works in intensive care medicine.

Meta-discourse – meta-discourse refers to a form of talk that operates at increasingly higher levels of generality and abstraction. Meta-discourse is the means with which actors identify and name the most central and most-likely-to-recur features of events and activities. The answer to the question, 'how do we do things around here?', may be meta-discursive: 'we always meet at 7, consult the notes, night staff hand over to day staff . . .' A critical aspect of meta-discourse is that it shifts away from specificity ('night staff gave the motor vehicle accident patient too much morphine during the night'; 'that nurse told both the consultant and the patient about the problem'), towards generality ('patients can be given morphine doses that are too high'; 'here, nurse clinicians can and will advise consultants and patients about incidents'), and abstraction ('a morphine overdose'; 'an incident disclosure'). Practitioners' developing a meta-discourse about their work is an integral component of their developing common ground, and this is the basis par excellence from which to organise and manage their work.

Passivity competence – this concept comes from Peter Sloterdijk's (2009) work where he discusses people's capacity for paying attention to events without reacting to them as one would normally. Not reacting to events means we keep our judgements and habitu-ated responses in abeyance. Paradoxically, passivity competence can expand people's capacity for action and effectiveness in action. This is because passivity competence unhinges action from routine and habituated responses and understandings, opening action up to quite different, because *reflexive*, possibilities. The special affordance of passivity competence lies in the fact that delaying and interrupting normal, habituated reactions may enable actors to become sensitised to a greater array of impressions. Delay and interruption of habituated conducts may open up people's contact with affect, or their affective potential.

Recession – recession is a concept borrowed from Peter Sloterdijk's work, and for him it refers not to an economic trend but to individual people distancing themselves from their self- and identity-defining habits. Recession marks a person's rejecting and re-inventing their self-defining psychological and behavioural traits. Recession and secession (see below) are related notions. For Sloterdijk, secession and recession are two sides of the same coin. They are rapidly becoming defining features of and cap-abilities for twenty-first century people enmeshed in rapidly reconfiguring social and organisational networks and practices (Sloterdijk, 2009).

Responsibility – responsibility refers to an obligation on the part of individuals to answer for actions they initiated or were meant to monitor and supervise.

Secession – secession is a concept borrowed from Peter Sloterdijk's work, and it refers to people distancing themselves from their social background, their personal and social 'home base'. Secession can manifest as national or international migration, but also as adopting conducts and behaviours that are in tension with those defining of our original (background) social context.

Peripheral participation – this concept refers to Lave's (1993) phrase 'zone of peripheral participation', which itself is a variation on Vygotsky's 'zone of proximal development' (Vygotsky, 1986). These notions refer to how learners benefit from acting within zones where they can observe others who are better skilled than they, and where they can experiment with activities and safely learn from errors.

Phronesis – Aristotle defines phronesis in terms of its aim: 'the end is merely doing well' (cited in Flyvbjerg, 2001: 56). It is 'a true state, reasoned, and capable of action with regard to things that are good or bad for man [sic]'. Emphasising its practical and pragmatic dimension, and contrasting it with scientific knowledge (*episteme*) and artistic production (*techne*), Aristotle adds: 'We consider that this quality belongs to those who understand the management of households or states' (Flyvbjerg, 2001: 57). Phronesis can be defined as practical knowing or 'knowing how'.

Reflexive – a reflexive attitude is one that seeks to frame and orient what one does and says with reference to what others do and say, coupled to the intention to attune what one does and say to what others do and say in an ethical–pragmatic sense rather than a strategic–exploitative sense. Relatedly, the present discussion contrasts reflexivity with reflection by regarding the former as adopting a socialising and contextualising perspective on one's actions, and the latter as favouring an individualising and psychologising perspective on one's actions (Iedema, 2011).

Registrar – a registrar is a doctor in the last year(s) of their training and before qualifying as a consultant or general practitioner. In the NHS, there are specialty registrars (8 years in post-university training) and general practice registrars 5 years of post-university training).

Resident – a resident is a junior doctor in training, one to two years out of university (also referred to now in the NHS as a 'foundation doctor').

Senior House Officer – a senior house officer is a junior or trainee doctor in the second year (or later) of their specialty training. In the NHS, this term has now been replaced with the term specialty registrar.

Video reflexivity – video reflexivity (also referred to as video reflexive ethnography; Iedema *et al.*, 2006) refers to the practice of filming professionals at work and sharing with them the resulting footage with the aim of engendering discussion about their work. Video reflexivity is at the basis of *HELiCS* (Handover: Enabling Learning in Communication for Safety), a training resource enabling frontline clinicians to determine their clinical handover systematisation needs by scrutinising their own *in situ* handover communication practices (www.centreforhealthcom.org/helics/).

Weave of commitment – the phrase weave of commitment is used to refer to how people act out their mutual and shared commitments. We use the metaphor of cloth or fabric to reduce our reliance on the mental dimensions of shared practice, and foreground the material and dynamic aspects of practice: its collaborative warp and communicative weft.

Health care practice improvement from within

*The education of the new professional will reverse the academic notion
that we must suppress our emotions in order to become technicians . . .
We will not teach future professionals emotional distancing as a strategy for personal survival. We will teach them instead how to stay close
to emotions that can generate energy for institutional change, which
might help everyone survive.*

—Palmer, 2007, cited in Berwick, 2009: w562

Preamble

In this chapter, we do the necessary groundwork to scaffold the main argument
of this book: people at the clinical front line are a critical source of insight and
momentum for dealing with the rising levels of complexity of care. This rise in
complexity is our first concern.

Vignette 1.1 Managing emergency department resources

One Monday morning, halfway through the school holidays, the emergency department of a large metropolitan teaching hospital was beginning to get busy. Very
quickly, patient demand began to outstrip the capacity of the department. Staff
were trying to cope as best as possible, inventing temporary solutions within the
emergency department and expediting the transfer of patients to other areas of the
hospital. When all the acute beds were occupied, staff began to locate a number of
patients in transitory assessment areas for stable patients, or 'cubes'.

> Lisa, a patient who was waiting for assessment and care, had been brought in by ambulance after becoming short of breath and feeling generally unwell. An older woman, Lisa had been to the emergency department before and was familiar with delays in care.
>
> Karen, the senior nurse unit manager, had joined her colleagues to assist in Lisa's clinical assessment and the initiation of treatment. Karen began Lisa's assessment in the corridor of the emergency department, near the ambulance bay. After some questions about why Lisa had been brought in to the emergency department and about her medical history, Karen did some initial clinical observations (pulse, blood pressure, temperature). She chatted a bit more with Lisa about how she felt, and about what might need to happen next. All through this, Karen was looking intently at Lisa. Then she said, 'I'll be back in a second.' She walked over to a senior doctor and said:
>
> *Karen:* Lisa is complex, she is going to hold cubes up.
> *Senior doctor:* Yep.
> *Karen:* So we need to put her here, in the corridor near the centre of the unit.
> *Senior doctor:* Yep, sounds good.
>
> Karen then walked back over to Lisa to explain she would be looked after not far from the nursing station and where Karen could easily see her.

The clinician at the centre of this vignette, Karen, is engaging in a complex manoeuvre. While chatting with Lisa, the patient, and glancing at the accompanying notes, Karen computes these and other less obvious issues into a calculation of the resources she is likely to have available. Risking the unit's ability to respond to other patients' needs, she decides that Lisa is to be granted special attention close to the observation desk, thereby taking up both scarce staff and scarce space resources. Her decision seeks to effect safety: she intuits Lisa's potential need for speedy medical attention, and she prioritises Lisa's needs, while trying to anticipate the implications of this decision for the unit's restricted resources and unpredictable rises in demand.

The vignette thus portrays emergency department clinicians collaborating and focusing on a complex task. The patient in question here may be sicker than is apparent, and may therefore need to remain close to the central observation desk. The additional uncertainties that complicate this brief event are multiple: there is uncertainty about how many beds the department will need; about access to medical staff in addition to the doctors who are currently present; about the speed with which patients can be referred on to other specialties; and about how many more ambulances and patients will arrive to call on the department's resources and services.

At the heart of the vignette, we find clinicians having to accommodate many competing issues at once: someone's sense that a patient may be sicker than is apparent and may possibly be in need of careful monitoring, an increasingly busy department creating uncertainty about bed numbers and staffing levels, and a lack of control over the speed with which patients are transferred to other specialties (Nugus *et al.*, 2010). The clinician's decision works for now, but it may need to be revisited when the next ambulance comes in. In that regard, decisions are made in the knowledge that the information currently available may be wrong or short-lived, that there may be additional information coming in that has significant implications for decisions made, and that new compromises and solutions may need to be devised at any moment. This requires them to 'think on their feet', showing resilience in the face of constantly changing circumstances (Wears *et al.*, 2008). In these ways, uncertainty creates complexity.

The kinds of complexity just described permeate how clinicians do their work, and they are integral to how they manage the quality and maintain the safety of patient care. Yet, these aspects of clinical work are rarely explicitly addressed in quality and safety discourse – whether characterising research, policy, or education and training. However, as we will argue, it should be precisely these wicked problems, tragic choices and dynamic complexity that need to be the focus of research and education if these are to have anything to say about how to accomplish quality and safety *in situ*.

We will introduce this argument in the following way: first, we will briefly discuss the dominant way of solving the problem of complexity and uncertainty, and point to its shortcomings (*see* next section, 'Current approaches to practice improvement: faith in knowledge and the known'). Then we will explain the relevance of a focus on *in situ* practices and introduce our approach, which we refer to as 'exnovation' (*see* 'A focus on *in situ* practice', p. 8). Then we provide an explanation of the aims of this book (*see* 'Aims of the book', p. 13). Towards the chapter's conclusion, we will present an outline of the chapters that are to follow (*see* 'Organisation of the book', p. 16). This enables the reader to decide whether to delve into the literature informing and supporting the approach presented here (Chapters 2–4), or whether to start looking at the various practical examples (Chapters 5–8).

Let us start, then, by taking a closer look at the resources currently made available to clinicians to cope with complex tasks.

Current approaches to practice improvement: faith in knowledge and the known

Generally the emphasis in clinical practice improvement is on expanding the scope of what *is* known (namely, 'filling knowledge gaps'). Such emphasis is suitable in situations that are simple and where processes are linear, sequential and repeatable. Here, a finite amount of knowledge is needed to explain what is going on. Treating the clinical work as if it were mainly and essentially linear, sequential and repeatable, practice improvement discourse highlights the importance of strengthening our control over the technical, managerial and proceduralisable aspects of work.

This perspective also informs most of the practice improvement approaches and methods deployed by health service researchers, on the understanding that the 'objects' under investigation or subject to intervention must remain strictly circumscribed, and that the results of such investigation are to be commensurable with the study's original points of departure. These constraints are realised by isolating selected aspects of 'the real'[1] for investigation (say, incident classifications and rates; subjects' responses to prefigured questions), by making available only certain discourses for framing the results, and, most critically, by radically divorcing the investigators' process of learning and discovery from that of the subjects (or objects) under investigation. In these ways, prevailing methodologies and pedagogies impose boundaries that help them circumvent, or, alternatively, deny them the complexities of the problems, choices and dynamics that confront clinicians in daily practice.

The resources that are made available to clinicians to cope with complex tasks, such as protocols, guidelines or organisational response charts (forms assisting staff with determining whether patients are deteriorating and are in need of specialised attention), are too often assumed to fit naturally into existing practice and its context. Of course, these resources need to be appropriately designed and potentially adapted to ensure uptake by local practitioners and sites. Here, context is critical. However, this means, at best, that the specific individuals,

---

1 We use scare quotes here ('the real') to flag that reality is not some unproblematic entity or set of entities 'out there'. We explain this point in greater detail in Chapter 3.

local sites and unique patient cohorts remain 'contextual' to the imperative of implementing rules and resources devised by 'experts elsewhere'. The principle here is that if we understand local contexts and their needs, we can heighten the chance that experts' rules and formalised resources are appropriately implemented (Ovretveit, 2011).

As per definition, generalised rules and resources do not and cannot take everyday practical complexities into account (Berg, 1998; Berg *et al.*, 2000). They are constructed on the basis of general scientific evidence, experts' views and 'first principles'. As generalisations, they are also necessarily simplifications. Their application to what actually happens need therefore not be self-evident at all (Star, 1995; Suchman, 1987). Without downplaying their importance for providing structure and context to everyday practices, we are concerned that they lack critical support for clinicians in their effort to connect these rules and resources to complex events. This is because complex dynamic processes are not linear, sequential and repeatable. Here, no amount of knowledge or evidence, and no number of guidelines and protocols, will provide a complete and comprehensive view of the practical choices and dilemmas facing front-line clinicians.

Guidelines are not self-explanatory: an example

In recent years, policy reform in Australia has moved to position the disclosure of incidents to patients and their relatives as central to incident management. When an incident occurs and there is an undesirable outcome of the care given, not only is an investigation performed but also the incident is openly discussed with those harmed. The treating clinicians or their managers may initiate the discussion, depending on severity, clinician confidence, and the level of formality and seniority deemed appropriate and/or expected by the person harmed and his or her relatives. A disclosure standard or guideline has been in force in Australia since 2003. State ministers agreed adoption of the principles promoted by the standard into state policy in 2008.

In response to questions about whether they practised disclosure, clinicians found it difficult to respond in terms of yes or no. The most frequently used response was 'it depends' (Iedema *et al.*, 2008). When interviewing patients and their relatives, we found a similar picture. Patients and relatives did not give yes or no answers to the question, 'Was your incident disclosed to you?' Instead, they told stories about complex, and at times conflicting, experiences. Some clinicians were open, others were more guarded; managers could be supportive or evasive; the process could go well one meeting and badly the next, and explanations could

---

swing from being satisfactory to being so technical as to not make any sense to them in relation to the original harm (Iedema *et al.*, 2011). Further interviews with clinical, quality and safety and managerial personnel about regulatory issues revealed a frequent lack of understanding or misunderstanding on the part of clinicians of the law surrounding disclosure (Studdert *et al.*, 2010). In sum, the guideline and then the policies available on disclosure translated neither into clear understandings about disclosure nor into uniform practices around responding to clinical harm.

Further, it was evident that interviewees commented positively on disclosure role-play training as a way of testing their responses to angry patient-actors, and observing colleagues making unsettlingly familiar mistakes. There are now sophisticated training programmes (see the Queensland Patient Safety Centre's website) where practising disclosures in the presence of trusted colleagues and actors provides a context for the nurturing of practical skill and confidence (Iedema *et al.*, 2009b). Such practice is critical to clarifying policy and translating knowledge ('knowing-that') into doing ('knowing-how'), and preparing practitioners for the communicative complexities that may lie ahead when they are called on to do incident disclosure.

Our preoccupation with general rules and formal resources has led to a dearth of strategies for tackling the more complex challenges of everyday work. To apply those rules and resources to situations replete with uncertainty and complexity, a mode of knowledge is necessary that is different from formal knowledge. What is needed is *practical* knowledge, or perhaps even practical knowing, to emphasise its dynamic nature (Nicolini, 2011). Their practical knowing determines whether clinicians are able to deploy general rules and resources 'on the run' in circumstances of uncertainty and complexity.

This practical knowing goes well beyond applying rules and resources. Clinicians make quality and safety decisions on a moment-to-moment basis, as shown by Karen in the earlier vignette. Equally, effective clinicians can handle *pervasive* uncertainty and complexity. They may be conscious of a whole range of unpredictable predictables, such as emergency call-outs or an excess of ambulances delivering very sick patients (Carroll, 2009). While junior clinicians may encounter what they experience as 'unpredictable unpredictables' – situations that call for expertise and solutions that are beyond their capability – senior practitioners are problem-solvers and risk-takers who do not shy away from bricolage and experimentation to counter and resolve problems (Jorm, 2012). As 'natural decision makers' (Klein, 1999), these practitioners may have an uncanny sense of how to get around challenges: they are able to generate the 'knowing' necessary for coping and succeeding (Mesman, 2008).

To achieve such levels of practical sophistication, Kahneman and Klein point out, the circumstances within which practitioners operate should not be overly complex. If circumstances are *way* too complex, the problem is not just that people's actions will be ineffective but also that they are denied the chance to learn from their ineffective actions (Kahneman and Klein, 2009). For them, learning can only take place amidst *moderate* levels of uncertainty and complexity – levels that are attuned to practitioners' own comfort levels.

Kahneman and Klein's argument may be true, but it takes for granted the notion that practitioners have only their own intelligence and knowledge to rely on when faced with uncertainty and complexity. For these commentators, practitioners are strangely isolated actors whose learning and actions are presented as operating in social isolation – even as kinds of solipsistic computation (Kahneman and Klein, 2009; Klein and Baxter, 2006).

In practice, clinicians negotiate the uncertainties and complexities that permeate their work together. That is how they gain and expand their practical knowing.

While important, these shared negotiations are by no means the full story. This is because they generally remain ad hoc and intermittent. Instead, and to capitalise better on the power of practical and shared knowing, clinicians need to become involved in processes that get them to look at and talk about the uncertainties and complexities that are inherent in and common to their everyday work.

This involves, first, the ability to step back from and observe the work as it unfolds. Second, it requires the ability to listen to others. It requires attention to detail and specific events, talking together about those details and events, paying attention to others and to what worries them, and re-articulating what clinicians think they know in order to share it, test it and revitalise it. A critical ingredient here is stopping what you are doing in order to see and listen. In Chapter 4 we return to discuss this critical behavioural manoeuvre. There we explain the significance of Peter Sloterdijk's notion of 'passivity competence' (Sloterdijk, 2009): the competence that is necessary for observing what is going on, becoming attentive, and listening to people and events around us.

This book provides examples of groups of clinicians who have taken the time to develop this competence and to deploy it. As the examples show, clinicians will target different aspects of their work, depending on what they find important, troublesome or fixable. The examples have in common that their reflexive orientation and their 'passivity competence' produce a shared intelligence. That is, through taking the time to observe their work and talk about it, practitioners develop a shared ability to question the taken-as-given, and a shared sense of what are the main opportunities and challenges. All this starts with focusing on 'the here and now', or on practice as it unfolds *in situ*.

A focus on *in situ* practice

Our focus in this book is on what clinicians do *in situ*, on the moment-to-moment unfolding of their practices. It is always intriguing to see how clinicians are inclined to take the moment-to-moment unfolding of their work for granted. They take it for granted on the assumption that they know what is happening. What they see as important instead is ready-to-hand information – people's assessment of the patient, the medical chart, and 'objective' data such as statistics, graphs, charts. What we want to do in this book is to say, bear with us, let's take some time to look at how practice unfolds and how are things done, from moment to moment, in the here and now. How do you do things, from moment to moment. Let's film it, let's describe it as a narrative, let's view it through the stories of patients. Let's *experience* it.

It turns out that, when clinicians consent to be involved, they are invariably fascinated by the resulting accounts and footage. This is, we believe, because they are confronted with what is deeply familiar, but in a way that renders it surprising and somewhat strange. The coupling of familiarity with surprise is what sparks their fascination. They see what they had taken for granted in a new light, from a new angle.

There is also a second reason for this fascination. For practitioners the footage or the narratives are not just about the few moments in time that are shown or talked about. Instead, they experience what they see and hear as *hologrammatic*; that is, a small piece of footage provides entry into large tracts of their working life and practical experience.

Put differently, what is visible and audible (the above-water part of the metaphorical iceberg) is complemented by practitioners' deep familiarity with what they see and hear (the iceberg's below-water part). The footage and narratives[2] spark knowledge of the scenes portrayed – of the histories that inform those scenes. They also engage the observer or listener at an affective level – they are

---

2   These narratives of course may be practitioners' stories or patients' and relatives' stories.

conscious of how it *feels* to be doing what those in the footage or the story are doing. In that way, what is seen and heard accrues richness and complexity. In that sense, video or narratives do not concern specific moments in time or specific people; on the contrary, they offer occasions for re-experiencing the complexities and rich dynamics of *in situ* care.

By replaying the complexities that confront clinicians in everyday practice in these ways, we seek to do more than just produce evidence of the ability of 'ordinary' clinicians to handle complex processes with resourcefulness and resilience. This book will show how clinicians will produce both ad hoc and *designed* solutions to address problems arising from the pervasive complexity of their work. *In situ* practice harbours a huge potential for innovation that originates from within practice, and this becomes evident when we take the time to consider what clinicians do – *especially* the specific activities and reasonings that they themselves engage in. However, to mobilise this potential, we need to observe and listen to what goes on, *in situ*.

As we will demonstrate in this book, observing and listening to what goes on *in situ* harbours enormous potential. Doing so can strengthen people's shared capacity for acting amidst complexity. It can also engender confidence in their ability to identify how to (re)design care processes. Observing and listening are the ingredients par excellence for realising patient safety from the bottom up, because they both manifest and nurture front-line practitioner intelligence. In later chapters we will talk about the skill to observe and listen using Peter Sloterdijk's notion of 'passivity competence' (Sloterdijk, 2009) – the competence to stop, observe and listen. Alongside patient safety's concern with practitioners applying 'off-the-shelf' and 'what works' solutions, this competence resists applying solutions in favour of a critical stocktake, and a sense-making that acknowledges the constraints and affordances inscribed into local sites and processes.

To be sure, there is a lot of pressure on front-line staff already, and asking them to reflect on the everyday dimensions of their work can be seen as yet another impost on their time. Moreover, talking about work is not always experienced as *doing* work, and may be seen as gratuitous and superfluous. There may be ambulances cueing outside, patients to be transferred, nurses to be informed and consultants to be contacted. All that may be true. However, we contend, contemporary clinicians have no choice. Their organisations are now so complex that no number of rules or amount of evidence can ever guarantee quality and safety. Although rules and evidence form a critical *ingredient* of quality and safety (Timmermans and Berg, 2003), the critical determinant is their *realisation*. Realising rules and evidence is an ongoing practical accomplishment.

This ongoing accomplishment cannot be an unreflexive accomplishment. That would amount to following rules blindly. Rules and evidence may be relatively static (the constant updates of guidelines and scientific findings notwithstanding), but realising them requires constant attention to *in situ* local uncertainties affecting actions, decisions and outcomes (Mesman, 2008). These uncertainties necessitate ongoing communication about which rules apply, how they apply, whether they apply, and whether we need new rules (Iedema *et al.*, 2010).

Here, rules and evidence are not ignored, and neither are they applied unthinkingly. Instead, the uncertainty that is inherent in their application is mediated and perhaps resolved through constant communicating. In situ communicating is the means par excellence for addressing and responding to the complexity that permeates clinical work. The reason communication plays such an important role is that it is dynamic and rapid, and as such it affords speedy learning. This learning is not just about what rules and evidence apply, but *how* they apply, *why* and *when*. Such communication is critical amidst complexity because knowing everything in complex circumstances is unlikely, if not impossible.

Even for the most senior experts, practice remains deeply uncertain (Jorm, 2012). Learning, therefore, is central and ongoing. It is central to safety, and it is central to the approach promoted in this book. However, we are concerned with learning of a special kind. We gloss it using the term *exnovation* (De Wilde, 2000). In contrast to *innovation*, which mobilises inventions produced by experts elsewhere and applies these to practice, exnovation expresses the principle that practitioners themselves already have resources that are critical to quality and safety, but that those resources need to be revealed, 'let out of the box' – not innovated but *ex-novated*.[3] Exnovation posits that clinicians share (or are able to share) a unique and constantly evolving practical wisdom. Exnovation emphasises that this wisdom needs to be *uncovered*, and *legitimated*, to clinicians themselves as much as to other stakeholders in care. It needs to be made explicit, nurtured, communicated.

But how do we 'exnovate'? Exnovation means involving front-line staff in articulating knowledge about and practical solutions for health care and clinical practices. In later chapters we will explain how to use this approach as a critical means to improving the quality and safety of health care. For now, we provide a brief overview of how it works. First, exnovation espouses a very specific educational philosophy. This philosophy states that people engage with the world, their

---

3   Exnovation can be considered as aggregation of 'excavation' and 'innovation'. Excavation has a double meaning, as it refers to 'exposure' of what is already there, as well as to 'digging out'.

work and themselves not principally through cognition or emotion but through shared *habits* (Dewey, 1922). Our habits are rarely fully conscious. Perhaps more contentious is the view that they are rarely purely individual. This philosophy regards most habits as *socially* promulgated and maintained. That is, we tend to do what others do, not least because that ensures our acceptance and legitimation.

Exnovation defined

Exnovation seeks to foreground the actual and potential richness hidden in everyday activity and front-line staff. Jessica Mesman has referred to exnovation as *highlighting* and *harnessing* 'the ecological strength of existing practices' (Mesman, 2007). Defined in that way, exnovation foregrounds and brings out what clinicians are already doing. Exnovation makes clinicians aware of their own existing ways of acting, and of their potential for change and expansion. In giving front-line clinicians confidence in the notion that their own practices are worthy of close attention, they gain in agency and control over existing process routines and outcomes. Exnovation involves asking the question, how do front-line practitioners cope from moment to moment? Asking this question enables us to probe how clinicians communicate and act in the here and now and also how doing so enables them to make their work safe (Gherardi and Nicolini, 2002; Weick and Roberts, 1993). Here, ongoing mutual checking of activities and their consequences, and sharing of tasks and renegotiating of knowledge and plans, are foregrounded. This produces a kind of *intervision* among actors, and this is what enables team members to handle irregularities, uncertainties, unpredictabilities and problems (Dekker, 2005). Exnovation makes it possible to describe these phenomena, and it enables practitioners to more consciously capitalise on these dynamic and dialogic sources of safety.

When do we become aware of our habits? When our habits encounter obstacles they become problematic, and we are forced to reconsider and revise how we deal with practical situations. Our inability to continue 'as was' generates energy, affect, emotion or (to use Dewey's term) impulse. For Dewey, changing our habits is only possible if there is sufficient impulse. Reasons, information, arguments and data are not enough to change habits. Change occurs when we become *affectively* implicated in a problem and in its solution.

> Concrete habits do all the perceiving, recognizing, imagining, recalling, judging, conceiving and reasoning that is done. (Dewey, 1922: 124)

So, habits can be changed, but not simply through thought. That is, we cannot consciously *will* our habits to change (Duhigg, 2012). We cannot *think* ourselves into new ways of acting, any more than we can whistle for wind (Dewey, 1922). Change involves us at the level of conduct and the body: we don't so much know how to act differently, as that we need to *sense* it, feel it in our bodies (Shusterman, 2008).

For that very reason, exnovation confronts clinicians with how they conduct themselves from moment to moment as living and feeling bodies moving in and through the world. While stories can provide important momentum, the medium par excellence for achieving this depth of engagement with how we conduct ourselves in practice is through videoing ourselves and viewing the resulting footage. The moving image confronts us with dimensions of practice that only drama and role-play may be able to replicate: How do we come across to others? What affective responses do we incur in colleagues and patients? What aspects of practice have we taken for granted, and what have we always considered as the most important, and why?

Footage such as this alerts us to all kinds of 'contextual' features – things and sentiments we tend to take for granted because in the 'real world' they are relegated to what surrounds us, the space of the taken-as-given. Because it reconfigures background and foreground, video footage enables us to see what happens in new ways. It teaches us to appreciate how we collaborate with others and thereby discern new possibilities. By viewing our shared practices, we allow footage to engender a shared awareness of the complexity in which we find ourselves and to which we are all subjected.

Our last point for now is that the effect of viewing video footage goes well beyond enhancing 'situational assessment and awareness' (Endsley, 2004). Situational assessment targets the risks and opportunities embedded in unfolding events, leading to situational awareness. For its part, exnovation engenders awareness on two different fronts: (1) it is embodied and affective (not simply cognitive) and (2) it is creative with respect to longer-term practice design (not just *in situ* problems and challenges requiring immediate resilience). It follows that exnovation is not just about retrospective analysis or prospective planning, but in the first instance about sense-making of 'what is' (Weick, 1995).

As the means to kick-start and explicitly articulate our sense-making, exnovation is something practitioners do together and experience together. Critical here is that observing oneself acting within a group brings out not so much who I am or how I act (although that is certainly part of it), but particularly who *we* are and how *we* act and relate as a social group. The video footage reveals us in our *social* dimension, how we are connected through activities, meanings and feelings – that dimension of what we do and who we are that patients sense when they walk into our unit or department (Langewitz, 2007). This is like when we walk into a dinner party and 'sense' the atmosphere within a split second of hearing people's voices and seeing their postures, gestures and movements. This sense-making is deeply emotional and social – one that has remained in the background in health services research because we have favoured individuals and their reasonings as our units of analysis and attention, not social interaction and distributed cognition. Exnovation, therefore, is unique in revealing the interactions that define teams and groups. It thereby also foregrounds the capacities and change potential of teams and groups.

In sum, the *in situ* dynamics of daily health care practices act not only as a source of complexity and uncertainty, but also harbour the resources to cope with complexity and uncertainty. To access these resources we need exnovation, as exnovation makes these resources tangible and opens them up for conscious appropriation or intervention. In Section 1 (Chapters 2–4) of this book we will explain the details and theoretical background of this approach, and in Section 2 (Chapters 5–8) we provide project examples. However, before doing so, we complete this introductory chapter with a discussion of the aims of this book and an overview of the chapters to follow.

Aims of the book

Overall, this book has a twofold aim. First, in contrast to others concerned about safety, we want to concentrate on the mundane, everyday activities that fill the clinician's working day. We suggested earlier that these activities are rich in information. They provide a 'hologrammatic' view into the workings of the team, the unit and even the organisation. Second, we want to sit down with clinicians and reflect on these activities, because we know that clinicians rarely have the opportunity to do so. We suggested earlier that considering such seemingly unimportant activities can engender considerable energy, insight and learning for clinicians. This is precisely because clinicians themselves intuitively appreciate that these apparently mundane aspects of their work *are* important. Surprisingly, these everyday aspects have to date not been mined in the interest of enhancing patient safety and the quality of care. That, in total, is exnovation, the focus of this book – the social-science of making moment-to-moment complexity visible, speakable and (re)designable, by involving clinician and patient stakeholders.

More generally, this book wants to assist clinicians (and patients) in how they handle and understand complexity, and in how they can build their own safety capacity. We will discuss the practical need for and theoretical background of collaborative attention. We also provide examples of how clinicians have achieved collaborative attention. Collaborative attention means having the patience to be open – open to what colleagues are doing and saying, open to the implications of what they are doing and saying, and open to colleagues having questions about what is appropriate to do and say. This book provides insight into how collaborative attention is integral to fine-tuning and improving the clinical work. We show that the question, 'what do clinicians need to do to display such collaborative attention?' is answered differently by different teams.

This book is further concerned with explaining the rich potential of this new way of thinking about safety and service complexity. We explain how involving practitioners in addressing these matters reveals and nurtures emergent capacities: they appreciate they can make a difference to how handovers are done, to how units organise transfers, or to how they communicate with other institutions. Part of the explanation is that these capacities are important to enabling clinicians to reflect *in* action (Schön, 1983), *in situ*. These capacities are equally central to practitioners reflecting *on* action, post hoc. This book promotes the perspective that groups can – and should – reflect together, collaboratively, to nurture their reflection on/in action. This enables them to turn such attention into a routine, building on a shared discourse and a recurring focus of attention and commitment. We refer to this latter activity not as reflection, which we associate with a quite personal and distanced activity, but rather as *reflexivity*. The term *reflexivity* is used to highlight the social, dynamic, practical and creative dimensions of the processes at issue here (Iedema, 2011).

In the course of this book we question a dominant trend in patient safety research and policymaking: to disregard that which is already present in what practitioners currently do (Bate and Robert, 2003). We want to give prominence to *existing* sources of safety. These sources of safety remain present in what clinicians do, despite generally being unrecognised and underappreciated. Generally, thanks to managers' and policymakers' concern with problems and deficits, these sources of safety are taken for granted and are regarded as devoid of innovative potential. Often, this is because these sources generally remain invisible, even when they constitute a critical dimension of how the work is accomplished (Star and Strauss, 1999).

Once made visible, however, these sources of safety can reveal their potential to practitioners and researchers alike. Exnovation provides the means to do this.

It offers a pedagogy enabling practitioners to make these sources visible and tangible, and act on them (De Wilde, 2000). Embedded in its pedagogy, therefore, are two dimensions. One, a *descriptive* dimension: this renders explicit how practitioners order their complex practices. Two, an *interventionist* dimension: this short-circuits enquiry, analysis, sentiment, insight, practice and change.

To capture how safety in health care practices can be improved by a focus on what is already in place, we will concentrate on communicative practices and *in situ* interactions. For us, these relations and communications form the principal resource through which team members accomplish safety. This is not to deny the critical influence of the dimensions of technologies and contexts on quality and safety (Vincent, 2010). What practitioners do well can be scuttled by badly designed tools and spaces. Equally, however, well-designed tools and spaces are no guarantor for quality and safety. Ultimately, trying to optimally design tools and spaces is forever challenged by unacknowledged conditions and unintended consequences. Moreover, circumstances change, staff move on, habits intervene, and so forth. No system can be so ideal and perfect as to accommodate and compensate for all these perturbations, and obviate their detrimental effects on patients' safety.

As we will show in later chapters, whatever ergonomic excellence is designed into the contextual, technological and systems dimensions of practice only in a limited way determines what practitioners do. The world (and thus health care) is now too complex. No system can be designed such as to cater for all complexity.

A brief note on 'communication'

Communication is defined here more broadly than merely verbal talk. Communication includes the many means that staff use to share information: body signals, facial gestures, scribbles on paper, actions affecting machine settings, and body states. Communication is therefore also and critically about how practitioners *feel*: their intuitive sense of what is happening. For example, when a nurse intuits that a patient is 'going downhill', or when a consultant feels that a junior doctor is not attuned to the seriousness of a patient's condition, their sense of the situation is likely to be communicated quickly and intelligently – a mere nod or frown may give expression to a person's sense that something needs attention. The way these signals are negotiated acts as an indicator of what we will refer to as the group's or team's *intelligence*. This is because these near-enough intangible and seemingly unimportant aspects of communication are in fact critical to realising teamness, and are central, therefore, to achieving quality of care and patient safety.

This book starts from the view that safe practice has two meanings. It distinguishes technical safety from affective safety. Technical safety refers to medical technologies and knowledges being mobilised as they should (namely, 'doing the right thing right'). Affective safety refers to the people who populate clinical environments feeling safe. This includes clinicians and patients. This book argues that safe care is achieved not merely through established routines but also through intelligent and learning attitudes towards the work.

Only by being attuned to one another will people get to *know* one another, and through that, understand the purpose and importance of the various aspects of the work. The examples provided in the second part of this book show how different clinicians in different parts of the world have taken the time to observe and listen to each other, and thereby develop a language together for addressing the complexities and rapidly changing clinical circumstances in which they find themselves.

Organisation of the book

This book is made up of two parts. The first part (Section 1, Chapters 2–4) is oriented towards setting out the relevant arguments and theories. These chapters explain the pedagogic and methodological bases of exnovation. The second part is practical. Here we provide examples of clinical sites where exnovation has been put into action. For those not interested in the theoretical and methodological underpinnings of exnovation, the second part of this book (Section 2, Chapters 5–8) will be of greater interest. For those wanting to understand how exnovation interfaces with existing research approaches in quality and safety, social science and practice innovation, these chapters will be of special interest.

In Chapter 2 we elaborate why engaging with clinical work means engaging with complexity. Complexity is a term that enables us to refer to an event without presuming that it has only one particular kind of significance, meaning, cause or effect. Complex events embody many different meanings for people. Therefore, too, these events do not predetermine what will happen next in any simple way. For that reason, confronting complexity involves and necessitates learning. This means that practitioners need to engage in 'complexity thinking', and in 'complexity talking'. These activities are central to enabling practitioners to solve problems *in situ* and anticipate such problems, as well as redesigning their work to minimise the likelihood of such problems arising in the first place.

In Chapter 3, we explain that if practitioners need to engage in 'complexity thinking and talking' to do their work, we cannot afford to presume that studying safety can rely on 'simplicity thinking and talking'. Where science has for centuries promoted 'rigorous' (read: inflexible) methods, and celebrated the knowledge that these methods have produced, research delving into complex processes such as the maintenance of safety has had to turn to 'flexible' approaches and methods to handle complexity. Such approaches and methods also acknowledge the emergent nature of research practice and the often unpredictable sources of solutions. Most critically, such approaches and methods do not just target the production of safety solutions – since such solutions are likely to be short-lived – but the generation of safety intelligence and passivity competence among front-line practitioners.

In Chapter 4 we turn again to the philosophy, pedagogy and practice of video-based exnovation. This chapter emphasises that exnovation involves working with front-line staff on thinking about and articulating a discourse to describe their ways of working, and thereby enhancing the ability of both clinicians and researchers to think and talk about everyday ways of working. Observing how practitioners work is a critically powerful source of information. This is so because we do not just engage with what practitioners say they do, but also with how they go about doing what they do. There is an important difference between asking people what they do and relying on their answers on the one hand, and observing what people do on the other hand, because what people say and what they do may differ (Greatbatch *et al.*, 2001). This is brought out forcefully when we show practitioners footage of their own ways of working, and they are obliged to acknowledge and come to terms with the everyday unfolding of their activities at work.

This leads us into Section 2 of this book. Chapter 5 brings together two accounts of exnovation, comparing and contrasting outsider-researcher-led facilitation with clinician-led facilitation. The first account draws on the work by Katherine Carroll in Australia; the second presents work by Gordon Caldwell in the United Kingdom. Both mobilised video-based exnovation for the purpose of revisiting doctors' ward rounds. While their process dynamics differed, the approaches produced similar questions such as, 'how can junior doctors learn to integrate a lot of complex information and present it at ward round in an orderly way?' This confirms that exnovation need not be driven by outsider facilitators, and that an insider catalyst can be equally effective.

Chapter 6 describes Jessica Mesman's project undertaken in a Maastricht neonatal intensive care unit. Describing the practical constraints and challenges that come into play when doing video-reflexive work, this chapter touches on how neonatal intensive care unit professionals enact infection control, how they come to appreciate their own and one another's skills, and what they felt they needed to change. This chapter also shows how video may act as mediator and catalyst of tensions that people have not been able to articulate at work and which they now can express and address.

Chapter 7 describes the experiences of Liesbeth van Rensen, Bas de Vries and Cor Kalkman with exnovation across six hospitals in and around Utrecht, in the Netherlands. Each of the hospitals has its own unique story, but each nevertheless offers generalisable outcomes. A point made in this chapter is that the project steering committee was unable to agree on the minimal data set for post-operative handover. It was acknowledged that local sites needed to be given the opportunity to develop their own systems. Having been granted this opportunity, the six sites developed their own systems, paying close attention to the details of handover practice. Here, the sheer weight of evidence makes apparent how important it is for hospital teams to produce their own post-operative handover changes and solutions, because it enables them to accomplish rich, multilayered approaches to safety. Indeed, this chapter puts on record the breadth of Utrecht's Patient Safety Centre video-reflexive achievements, showing the power of team-based 'complexity thinking-talking'.

Chapter 8 describes a Sydney-based project that targeted the communication process between ambulance officers and triage nurses in emergency departments. By filming these handovers, analysing them, and involving paramedics and emergency clinicians in debate over what kind of information would be appropriate to be included in a protocol, participants were able to develop a set of information items critical to both paramedics and nurses. The project involved rapid feedback training in the new protocol, as well as a video-based evaluation analysis of the redesigned handover practice. The results of the research have now been integrated in the New South Wales Ambulance curriculum, as well as being made available to all emergency departments around the state of New South Wales on a DVD and via a weblink.[4]

Chapter 9 concludes the book. In this chapter we summarise the implications of this new improvement paradigm for health services research. In doing so, we articulate a new agenda for patient safety and quality of care research that encompasses not merely what clinicians know but how they structure their relationships and team-based dialogues. We argue that this new paradigm is critical for obviating what Dekker refers to as organisations' 'drift into failure' (Dekker, 2011).

---

4   See www.archi.net.au/resources/safety/clinical/nsw-handover/ambulance-ed

Section 1

2

The complexity of health care work

Introduction

Health care work is becoming increasingly complex. This complexity arises in part from the difficulties clinicians have in determining what is wrong with patients, and from uncertainties about how care is to be organised across team, specialty and department boundaries (*see* Box 2.1).

Box 2.1 An avoidable urinary tract infection

Marissa had a severe urinary tract infection. She still had a fever and fast pulse after 24 hours of intravenous antibiotics. The medical team saw her on Friday and noted she could go home on Saturday on oral antibiotics if her fever settled, without seeing a doctor. Her fever settled, but she was not discharged, presumably because this decision was not appropriately communicated or documented. By Monday she had a cannula site infection needing another antibiotic. Then she needed a deep vein thrombosis test DVT because the medical team in charge then forgot to start dalteparin. She subsequently developed a pulmonary embolism and hospital-acquired pneumonia. She had to be admitted to the intensive care unit, where she had a tension pneumothorax on the ventilator, suffered some brain damage, and also developed *Clostridium difficile* diarrhoea. This cascade of incidents produced a number of incident reports, a root cause analysis of the *C. difficile*, and an out-of-court settlement for the failure to discharge on the Saturday and for all the subsequent hospital-acquired harm.

Perhaps if Marissa's medical team had communicated their Friday ward round decision more effectively and the weekend team had discharged her as expected, no extra care would have been needed for this patient, no time would have been spent on writing incident reports, no effort would have been put into doing a root cause analysis, and no money would have been spent on the out-of-court settlement. Marissa's case is an example of how problems can rapidly escalate. Perhaps clinicians on duty on the Saturday felt the fever had not settled sufficiently. However, their decision (or perhaps their oversight) not to discharge Marissa produced disastrous consequences for her, for her clinicians, and for the hospital. Obviously, these kinds of complexities are difficult if not impossible to anticipate, even if they may seem simple to explain with the benefit of hindsight (Wears and Nemeth, 2007).

Not discharging Marissa may have resulted from a related source of complexity that practitioners are (or should be) generally better able to anticipate and address: clinicians espousing very different views on what are the best approaches to patient treatment.

Box 2.2 In-specialty disagreement about treatment standards

Necrotising enterocolitis (NEC) is a devastating inflammatory disease of the gastrointestinal system that is common in very premature infants. Every single day, clinicians in the neonatal intensive care unit (NICU) assess the small bodies of the premature babies for NEC, and watch for any early warning signs and symptoms of the disease such as blood in the stools, abdominal distension and gastric residuals after feeds. The appearance of NEC is dreaded by neonatologists, as it is associated with significant morbidity and mortality and prolonged hospitalisation and as a result it creates a large cost burden on the NICU and the health system at large of between USD$20 000 and $75 000 per case.

However, NEC has a complex and multifactorial aetiology in addition to a broad spectrum of presenting symptoms. This makes NEC prevention, early detection and diagnosis difficult. Despite decades of NEC research, only small gains have been made in finding the causes and treatments of NEC. Recent research reveals that an exclusive breast milk diet for premature infants (instead of a diet that includes bovine-based infant formula) is a successful way to reduce rates of NEC. Consequently, many NICUs throughout the world promote a diet of breast milk. This means that when a mother's own breast milk is unavailable, donated breast milk is promoted as an alternative to formula in order to prevent NEC. However, in the United States donor milk is not covered by health insurance and so the cost of donor milk at USD$3.50 per ounce is passed on to parents or absorbed by the hospital. Consequently, in some hospitals donor milk is not made available to infants or, alternatively, parents are required to pay for it.

A US NICU was reviewing their policy of providing donor milk at a cost to parents. At the policy meeting, neonatologists discussed a potential change to hospital policy that would make donor milk available to all babies in need at no cost to the parents. The following discussion between three neonatologists reveals the way conflicting truths about the cause of NEC impact on the delivery of health care.

Neonatologist 1: I am a believer in the evidence of breast milk preventing NEC. If we supply donor milk free of charge to parents, we will ensure every baby has access to breast milk, whether or not a mother can provide it. If we prevent just one case of NEC we would save enough money to pay for 2 years' supply of donor milk to the whole NICU!

Neonatologist 2: That's right. The cost of donor milk is a drop in the bucket in relation to the total cost of the baby's stay here in the NICU.

Neonatologist 3: I need to play devil's advocate. There is not sufficient evidence that an exclusive breast milk diet prevents NEC, so I believe any extra money should be put towards assisting mothers to breastfeed, rather than to provide free donor milk.

Neonatologist 1: As you can see, not all neonatologists are on the same page about NEC prevention and the role of breast milk. However, we need to examine the cost-benefit analysis of providing donor milk to the most vulnerable babies if they cannot receive their mother's own milk.

The example provided in Box 2.2 indicates that scientific evidence, clinical treatments or care philosophies need not be self-evident, straightforward or shared. This means that complexity is not merely produced by illness and disease but also by how clinicians and health care services structure their responses to clinical matters.

To explain the different aspects of complexity, we first refer to the categorisation proposed by Lillrank and Liukko (2004), as that categorisation helps us explore the dimensions of safety (*see* next section, 'Levels of complexity and conditions for safety'). That discussion leads us into consideration of what makes for an effective team, and the proposition that here communication and learning play a major role (*see* 'Team health and group effectiveness', p. 29). This is, as we will show in the section 'Safety in/as practice: making sense of complexity'

(p. 34), because communication and learning form the bases of adaptive behaviour, as they offer ways of coping and acting with complexity. We conclude this chapter (*see* 'The role of front-line intelligence in group collectivity', p. 38) with a summary of why people's *in situ* conducts are criterial for team effectiveness and patient safety. We also discuss how effective conducts can be learned and shared.

Levels of complexity and conditions for safety

For Lillrank and Liukko, the complexity of clinical work can be broken down into three levels (Lillrank and Liukko, 2004). At the 'standard' level, the work is made up of mainly identical and repetitive activities. Here we can think of how a ward or room is cleaned, or how surgical instruments are autoclaved. If something untoward happens this is likely to be due to a lack of procedural compliance, and this will manifest as a 'deviation' from established practice (*see* Figure 2.1).

At the 'routine' level, the next level up, activities are similar but may not be entirely identical. Here, activities are enacted according to a guideline or a protocol. Unlike procedures, guidelines tend to be slightly more abstract and general, allowing somewhat more decision-making discretion but within strict limits. Here we can think of a nurse or junior doctor handover that follows the SBAR protocol (a handover protocol that structures information as situation, background, assessment and recommendation). Actors have discretion over how to flesh out the different handover components, but not including one of them (e.g. not providing a treatment recommendation) may be regarded as inappropriate, or even as an error.

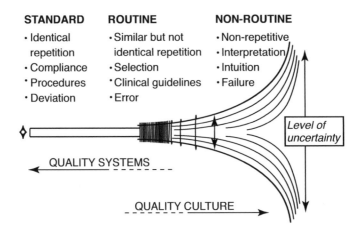

FIGURE 2.1 The quality broom

The third level of complexity is 'non-routine'. Here, uncertainty is quite pronounced, and decision-making is contingent on numerous factors requiring actors to use their interpretation and intuition. At this level, procedures, guidelines and protocols may still apply, but contradictory signs, incomplete information, conflicting interpretations and competing interests may confound their rules and advice. If a decision here produces an unexpected outcome, it may be regarded as a failure.

Lillrank and Liukko's schema is attractive in that it explains the different dimensions of safety. Safety is not uniform: it assumes different guises at different levels of complexity. Standard processes are best enacted with *compliance*, routine processes are best enacted on the basis of *adherence*, and non-routine processes demand creativity, or what we may refer to as *emergence*. In short, some clinical work processes require more clinical experience, creative thinking and professional competence than others. This is particularly the case when competing 'safeties' are at work, such as when a trade-off needs to be achieved between lowering the risk of infection and deploying a reusable device (rather than a non-reusable device) that may not be fully sterilisable but that is easier to handle because it is less rigid. Here, delicate decisions come into play about whether device flexibility outweighs infection risk (Rowley, 2011). It also seems clear that these levels of complexity are unlikely to manifest on their own, or discretely. Rather, events are more likely to be made up of all three levels to a greater or lesser degree, with some level(s) being more prominent than others at different times.

Hence, events will be multilayered – they are likely to encompass both simple and complex dimensions, and only selected aspects of what happens are likely to be fully iterative, routine or non-routine. This last point has important implications for how we understand the accomplishment of patient safety. Two implications stand out.

1. Multilayered events require teams of practitioners whose collective skills, training and experience enable them to handle and manage such events' entire range of iterative, routine and non-routine dimensions.
2. Team members have to continually ensure that their skills, training and experience are optimal and complementary to enable them to effectively handle and manage the full range of actual and potential complexities.

These two implications are central to the concerns of this book, and they are the backdrop for the change and improvement pedagogy promoted here. Basically, our thesis is that the complexity of everyday events necessitates front-line practitioner involvement in the resolution of problems – not just the resolution of here-and-now problems pertaining to specific patients or even cohorts of patients, or the resolution of problems arising from how to apply a rule or a guideline or a checklist, but the resolution of problems to do with the suboptimal organisation of patient care, with patients' negative experiences of such care, and with practitioners' conflicting assumptions about that care.

Too often patients find themselves in care, witnessing a lack of team communication, interprofessional conflict, cross-departmental rivalry, and a general lack of organisational acumen. For good reason, this does not inspire confidence.

Is following rules safer than relying on intuitive expertise?

Kahneman and Klein address the question of whether 'following rules is safer than relying on intuitive expertise' (Kahneman and Klein, 2009). In answering this question, they reason as follows. The determination of whether intuitive judgements can be trusted requires an examination of the environment in which the judgement is made and of the opportunity that the decision-maker has had to learn the regularities of that environment. Task environments are 'high-validity' if there are stable relationships between objectively identifiable cues and subsequent events or between cues and the outcomes of possible actions. An environment of high validity is a necessary condition for the development of skilled intuitions. Other necessary conditions include adequate opportunities for learning the environment (prolonged practice and feedback that is both rapid and unequivocal). If an environment provides valid cues and good feedback, skill and expert intuition will eventually develop in individuals of sufficient talent. Although true skill cannot develop in irregular or unpredictable environments, individuals will sometimes make judgements and decisions that are successful by chance. These 'lucky' individuals will be susceptible to an illusion of skill and to overconfidence. Intuitive judgements can arise from genuine skill and be accurate but they can also arise from inappropriate application of heuristic processes and be wrong. True experts, Kahneman and Klein note, know when they don't know (but not why they know or not know). However, non-experts (whether or not they think they are) certainly do not know when they don't know. Subjective confidence is therefore an unreliable indication of the validity of intuitive judgements and decisions. What Kahneman and Klein term 'fractionation of skill' is another source of overconfidence. Professionals who have expertise in some tasks are sometimes called upon to make judgements in areas in which they have no real skill. Fractionation occurs in task environments such as medicine where routine diagnoses can be interrupted by uncommon case

---

presentations that are nevertheless regarded as calling for routine care. Finally, the authors argue that weak regularities available in low-validity situations can sometimes support the development of formal algorithms that produce better outcomes than chance. Think of examples such as the critical pathway and the clinical guideline, both offering prescriptions for action. These algorithms only achieve limited accuracy given practical variations, but they outperform individual human choice because of their advantage of consistency. However, the authors acknowledge that allowing algorithms to fully govern human action may have undesirable side effects (Kahneman and Klein, 2009), as in cases where a pathway was adhered to even though the patient's clinical problem and need exceeded the pathway in complexity.

As noted earlier, Kahneman and Klein's reasoning takes the individual, isolated actor as their point of departure. In health care, clinicians collaborate (or should collaborate on solving problems). The 'distributed' nature of what clinicians know and do has not really been investigated, even if it is referenced in terms like 'resilience' and 'mindfulness'. Video capture and exnovation bring these latter aspects to the fore: both foreground the quality of connectedness that exists among clinicians, and which bears on whether and how safe care becomes possible.

Working in low- to medium task-validity environments, clinicians often face sub-ideal conditions (Runciman *et al.*, 2007) – insufficient resources, understaffing, difficult patients, ageing technologies and equipment, unreasonable working hours, and so forth. Expecting clinicians to address these environment or 'system' problems may be beyond their power and influence (Amalberti *et al.*, 2005), particularly when the causes of these sub-ideal conditions are external. For example, think of the difficulties associated with treating chronically ill patients' co-morbidities in services where specialties operate more or less autonomously.

The causes for sub-ideal systems can also be internal, or self- and practice-induced – the interests of departments being put above those of patients, the complexities inherent in care being exacerbated thanks to disagreements being allowed to continue to complicate patient care. Here, think of the example given in Box 2.2: is human breast milk effective for limiting NEC or not? If clinicians have conflicting experiences of particular treatments, should they allow such differences to persist? In some instances, experimentation with different approaches may be fruitful, particularly if the outcomes of the different approaches are evaluated. In others, and where outcomes are not compared, variation may be dictated by blind habit, creating potentially unnecessary complexities and therefore dangers.

Now, let us summarise the discussion as follows.

- Teams of practitioners with various and different competencies are critical to enabling a service to confront the full range of demands and complexities likely to be inherent in care provision.
- Team members must regularly communicate about how their skills, training and experience complement one another, and about whether these are adequate (or are rendered adequate through appropriate training and supervision) for confronting the various task complexities they (may) face.
- The safety of care is contingent on the ability of clinicians to (discern whether they) collectively meet the standard, routine and non-routine aspects of clinical events.

Here, we have broadened the conventional notion of safety that stipulates that actions and decisions comply with scientific evidence and clinical guidelines. Safety also includes team members collaborating such that their skills, training and experience meet the full range of complexities they may face (Vincent, 2010). This may necessitate resilience (Hollnagel, 2006) and workarounds (Gasser, 1986). Workarounds of course may be so frequent and integral to the work that they are promoted to become formally part of practice. Lastly, safety further includes team members evaluating whether and how they are placed to meet these dynamic complexities and potentially revising how they should meet those complexities.

The patient safety literature spends much time deliberating the first of these conditions, and measuring whether clinical practice complies with existing evidence and guidelines (Mangione-Smith *et al.*, 2007; McGlynn *et al.*, 2003). Increasing attention is now devoted to the second of these conditions, thanks to important statements on front-line practitioner resilience (Hollnagel *et al.*, 2006), clinical micro-systems (Mohr *et al.*, 2004) and team communication (Lingard *et al.*, 2005, 2002).

The third condition, however, has received limited attention. Front-line clinicians are generally not regarded as *producers* of evidence, or of practical knowledge. They are the *executors* of knowledge and the *users* of evidence. There are of course exceptions to this. Recently, we have begun to hear about practice-based evidence, but here the emphasis is still on the production of formal and generalisable knowledge that is to be imposed again on others elsewhere (Horn and Gassaway, 2007). For its part, the 'collaboratives' initiative was groundbreaking in its attempt to harness front-line clinicians' insights to the cause of safety (Schouten *et al.*, 2008). However, some exceptions notwithstanding, collaboratives are often narrowly focused to address a medical-scientific question and their tasks are generally technically and not reflexively defined (Zuiderent-Jerak, 2007).

For their part, and while also a critical opportunity for front-line clinicians to articulate their practical knowledge, critical pathway initiatives aim to outline optimal ways of working by bringing front-line practitioners together in articulating the common contours of their work (Pinder *et al.*, 2005). However, here too the focus is on 'objective' aspects of the clinical work, rather than on the stakeholders themselves and the actual work they do together. In assuming this focus, pathway projects too often miss the opportunity to address team competence, team member communication and, more generally, the kind of 'team health' that is requisite for clinicians to take stock of how well they are placed to confront workplace complexity (Iedema, 2011). Before moving on to how people make sense of complexity, let us delve a bit deeper into the notions of 'team health' and 'group effectiveness'. As we will show, how people handle and intervene in their own 'habituations' plays an important role here.

Team health and group effectiveness

'Team health' and 'group effectiveness' (Cohen and Bailey, 1997) are now recognised as critical to safety. They point to appropriate collaboration and support among practitioners generally, and to appropriate supervision of and learning among novices (Lemieux-Charles and McGuire, 2006). A recent overview by Street *et al.* (2009) has comprehensively described the link between health and communication. Albeit writing from the patient's perspective, they regard effective and sensitive communication to have both indirect and direct health effects (*see* Figure 2.2). Indirectly, such communication produces proximal outcomes including understanding, satisfaction, agreement and trust. Intermediate outcomes include access to care, quality medical decision-making and commitment to treatment.

They define direct health outcomes to include survival, cure and remission, less suffering, (better) pain control, and the like (Benedetti and Amanzio, 2011). These improved health outcomes of communication for patients should translate into advantages for clinicians as well. Moreover, if communication has health outcomes for patients, the quality of communication among clinicians themselves of course also has health outcomes for *them*. Good communication may lessen the uncertainties faced by novices when dealing with complexity; it may obviate tensions among clinicians and clarify treatment decisions and simplify management plans; it may enhance a team's ability to handle multilayered clinical-organisational complexities, and it may position team members more advantageously when faced with entirely unpredictable events.

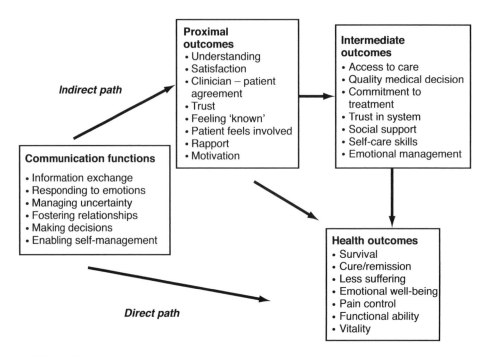

FIGURE 2.2 Direct and indirect pathways from communication to health outcomes

We now have many kinds of assessments of team health and group effectiveness. These include ones that assess team members' uptake of checklists as evidence of the quality of their 'information exchange and team cohesion' (Lingard *et al.*, 2005). Others evaluate teams' communication behaviours to determine their degree of professional collaboration or segregation (Finn, 2008). Some regard team communication as sufficiently linear for it to be profitably subjected to ran-domised trial conditions capable of revealing generalisable results (Zwarenstein *et al.*, 2009). Again others insist that communication is the domain where prac-titioners confront and negotiate complexity, thus lacking linearity and resisting predictability (Iedema and Merrick, 2012). Finally, team members' need to communicate in ad hoc ways about emerging information, unfolding situations and challenging problems has been found in some cases to produce undesirable and even dangerous interruptions (Alvarez and Coiera, 2005; Coiera and Tombs, 1998), and in others as manifesting a flexibility and adaptability that may be necessary amidst complexity (Iedema *et al.*, 2010).

These various findings and positions notwithstanding, the association between communication, team health and group effectiveness seems incontestable (Cohen and Bailey, 1997). But if communication is indeed the means by which practitioners articulate and negotiate complexity, it may therefore also be difficult or perhaps even undesirable to fully regulate it and proceduralise it. Evidence of improved communication leading to better patient outcomes has certainly been produced, and some of these interventions relied on simple checklists and protocols (Pronovost *et al.*, 2006). However, it is also acknowledged that checklists are unlikely to be the sole factor in improvement, and that the full story of how improvements are achieved is considerably more complex, involving intricate political, interpersonal and other manoeuvres and tactics for solutions such as a checklist to be considered worthwhile in the first place (Bosk *et al.*, 2009).

Rather than assuming that team health and group effectiveness can be simply invoked by instituting a checklist or a protocol, or thinking that team health and group effectiveness can be derived from some other kind of 'magic bullet', we should inquire into the pedagogic or learning conditions that may render the presence of team health and group effectiveness likely. For example, are front-line practitioners used to speaking about their day-to-day practices in personal, social and organisational terms, not just in technical-clinical terms (Iedema *et al.*, 2009a)? That is, do they have a discourse for speaking about how they work together, and what that work entails? When we consider team communication from this angle, it becomes apparent that practitioners often lack a discourse for addressing confounding issues and common concerns. They will also claim not to have the time to rehearse such discourse.

This lands us in a peculiar territory. When we probe these matters, the following puzzle presents itself. Staff are immensely knowledgeable about what they do, even many junior staff. They often have worked in a variety of care services and have experienced numerous ways of dealing with patients and diseases. At the same time, and paradoxically, they are not necessarily fully conscious of what they do from moment to moment, presumably because much of this is taken as given. We will return to this point in Chapter 4, but for now we restrict ourselves to the following observation.

As people who find themselves in clinical work situations day in day out, practitioners have, besides their conscious knowledge of how things work and experience of what happens on a specific day, a 'tacit' understanding of the logic of care, and of the opportunities for change within the framework of how they work. Why do junior medical doctors sit around the coffee table for their handover, without checking on patients together, and without writing anything down?

When we ask them, they'll say, 'because we are run off our feet, and this is the only time we have to catch our breath'. Is that a good enough reason? It will be if their training lacks consistent modelling of bedside ward rounds, denying them experience of their benefit for patient management. But once they've been asked the question, they may be reminded of how they sit there casually discussing patient issues over a coffee with someone typing information into a computer and others walking in and out, they may have been enabled to reflect on their own work. This may render them capable of intervening in what otherwise would persist as taken-as-given practice (Richmond *et al.*, 2011).

In asking practitioners this kind of question, something remarkable occurs: people who rarely have the opportunity to think about the general logic of their ways of working, suddenly turn out to be able to develop a language to describe their work processes. They are able to develop practice-relevant insights into information and responsibility exchange, patient safety and quality of care. This is because practitioners are not automatons, unthinkingly carrying out the practices they were trained into; they are thinking, cognate beings who have opinions about the effectiveness of their practices, and who are concerned – most of the time – to do well. Nor are they, as a rule, 'resistant' workers, persistently dismissive of health departmental strategies aimed at improving the outcomes of the work. If we want to find out about front-line staff's own insights, understandings and views on practice, then we need to take the time to talk to them and allow them to talk. Most important, we need to give them a view of where they are now, and how they are carrying out their work, from moment to moment.

Without involving practitioners in this way, the actual reality and full potential of existing work practices will remain largely invisible. They will remain invisible, even though front-line staff are embedded in these practices and live them on a day-to-day basis. In fact, it is precisely because front-line staff live these work processes on a day-to-day basis that they 'learn to forget' what these processes look and feel like, what their logic is, what their impacts are. This is *habituation*. Staff become habituated into having ward rounds at 7 a.m. and 5 p.m., without asking the kind of questions that may occur to outsiders such as patients, relatives and researchers: Why do you have 12 people standing around during a ward round, only four of whom can hear what is being said, and there is no dialogue or questioning of what is said because the senior consultant has already decided what needs to be done? Why is there only one person, and sometimes no one, taking notes? How can you concentrate on crucial information when those speaking do not raise their voice above the ward noise? Why do you have these ward rounds when the things that you are discussing may be superseded by new information before you have finished discussing them? Why do you not involve other professionals from the team in your ward round?

Habituation means that staff become not merely acculturated to 'how things are done around here' but also that staff learn to forget how to ask questions about 'how things are done around here'. This also means that they have learned to forget what kind of questions to ask (Dewey, 2004; Shusterman, 2008). Writing in the 1950s, Isabel Menzies-Lyth put these habituations and forgettings down to staff acculturating into ritualised ways of managing grief and anxiety in the face of disease, suffering and dying. She even saw clinicians' organisational habits as warding off staff resentment and envy of the care that patients receive (Menzies-Lyth, 1988; Skogstad, 2000). This perspective on how health care is structured regards the process of staff forgetting how to ask questions about how they conduct their work as motivated by irrational kinds of affect – specifically, negative feelings. We cannot confront the full extent of our fears or misgivings, so we lapse into 'irrational behaviours' and stop asking questions. Others who have commented on the apparently 'illogical' (non-patient-centred) way in which clinical practices are organised see their inertia and rigidity as motivated not by anxiety or envy but, rather, by the need to normalise existing political and interpersonal 'weaves of commitment' with which practitioners have identified and thus become implicated (Garfinkel, 1967).

These views on the ways in which services are organised are to a greater or lesser extent 'dystopian'. Dystopian means that there is limited hope for improving practice. This is because people are caught up in complex personal, interpersonal and organisational pathologies that are beyond their control and that inevitably compromise practice.[5] Despite their dystopian outlook, neither Menzies-Lyth nor Garfinkel lapse into 'deficit thinking' – thinking that regards practice as inherently 'faulty'. These theorists regard practice as harbouring a logic that, according to definition, does not easily map onto organisational structures and bureaucratic ideals. To expect practices to be linear, rational and fully rule-bound is to misunderstand their often arbitrary basis and logic (Bourdieu, 1990).

Now, the foregoing adds up to the following critical conclusion. The complexities of everyday work and interpersonal relationships – particularly in health care! – are best handled using the insights, intelligence and creativity of those who live and work amidst those complexities.

Admittedly, this raises the question of how clinicians actually make sense of

---

5   Isabel Menzies-Lyth acted as consultant to a number of organisations and sought to improve the way that employees organise their work, and she was able to report a number of improvements (Menzies-Lyth, 1988).

complexity. As we will show in the next section, making sense of and managing complexity are critically dependent on 'adaptive behaviour'. Making sense of complexity implies, then, that we need to make sense of our own and others' adaptive behaviour.

Safety in/as practice: making sense of complexity

From the industrial accident and organisational safety literature we know that practice is safe not just thanks to being systematised and mapped out in the form of procedures and guidelines, but also thanks to employees creatively and attentively adapting to day-to-day and moment-to-moment 'unpredictables' (Gherardi, 2007). These unpredictables include two types of events: (1) events that clinicians know can occur any moment ('unpredictable predictables') and, albeit less common, (2) events that people are entirely unable to predict ('unpredictable unpredictables') (Carroll, 2009).[6] The important point here is that, while guidelines, protocols and procedures are crucial to enabling staff to schematise and thereby prepare for what they do, such resources in and of themselves generally remain silent about how to connect to the lived experience of work, and therefore on how to handle unpredictables.

Rationalising how clinical work is done is crucial to enabling staff to 'make sense' of what they and others do (Weick, 1995). Rationalising clinical work means creating road signs: rules, protocols, and the like. Without road signs, we are likely to get lost, particularly in complex places like hospitals and health services. However, sense-making draws on more than signs, formal resources and rules alone. Sense-making relies on staff being able to have a dialogue about what is (un)predictable, how (un)predictable these events are, and what to do in response to such events.

One way in which the importance of dialogue to safety becomes evident is by considering how clinicians interact with each other in 'marginal spaces' such as corridors. When videoing corridor interactions, we found that apparently *ad hoc* and disconnected conversations played an important role in practitioners' accomplishment of safety (Iedema, *et al.*, 2010). Clinicians run into one another, and enter into unplanned conversations. These conversations can be highly disruptive (Coiera *et al.*, 2002). But, because these conversations are unconstrained

---

6   Of course, unpredictability inversely correlates with familiarity with the work, clinical seniority and work experience (Carroll, 2009).

by formalities like the ones that govern the case conference or the patient consult meeting, they also allow clinicians a high degree of conversational freedom.

When observed closely, this freedom turns out to enable clinicians serendipitously to address crucial issues. It allows them to raise issues that are foremost in their mind. As we showed in earlier research that draws on this data (Iedema, *et al.*, 2010), clinicians 'adaptively' orient to what becomes significant at the moment of their encounter (Kornberger and Clegg, 2004). They may shift dynamically and rapidly from issue to issue, or even consider multiple issues simultaneously.

Consider the dialogue shown in Vignette 2.1. Here, clinicians talk about two things at the same time: (1) the management of a pressure ulcer patient and (2) how to tie an infection control gown.

Vignette 2.1

Doctor: [He (patient) should not] sit up so much. He's sitting up for 6–8 hours.

Occupational therapist: How is the pressure area?

Doctor: It's a grade one area [*indicating size with fingers, not large*], but he's got no fat over his IT [ischial tuberosity] area, so he's going to have to be another couple of weeks off it, just to finish it off.

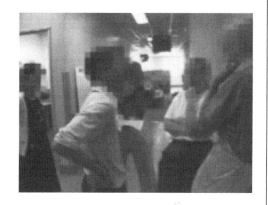

Occupational therapist: But he hasn't . . . [*tying apron around front*]

Nurse: [*reaching hand in occupational therapist's direction*] Don't tie it around the front.

Doctor: Yeah [*reaching hand out, smiling*] I can't do the back tie.

Occupational therapist: [*ties apron around the back*] He hasn't agreed to . . . um . . . any equipment or anything. He's not on a mattress, or anything. [*looking at clinical nurse consultant*] He's just on his own bed.

Let us consider what happens here. When seeing the occupational therapist, the spinal doctor is reminded of the spinal patient who had to be sent up to the intensive care unit (ICU). They discuss the inadequacy of the mattress the patient is likely to lie on in the ICU. As they tie on their protective gown (to visit a pressure ulcer patient potentially carrying an infection), their conversation shifts towards tying the gown on properly. The conversation then shifts back to the mattress. This short and apparently inconsequential sequence shows that safety is created not just by following procedures, or even just by adapting procedures to practical circumstances. The sequence shows that safety also results from clinicians being attentive to the unique way in which circumstances unfold in the present at different levels, and sometimes simultaneously. Here, several safety issues coalesce: a patient requiring a different mattress; a colleague tying their apron on inappropriately; a doctor advising a social worker; a nurse advising a doctor and a social worker.

The vignette shows how inventive and attentive front-line staff can be in their effort to enact safe practice. This example highlights one of the dimensions of clinical practice that this book is about: safety that emerges from staff being attentive and inventive in the here and now. This, we suggest, is 'the dark side of the moon' in so far as patient safety thinking is concerned. The other dimension that patient safety thinking and its focus on formalising practice tend to obscure is the potential for learning that is at the heart of being attentive and inventive. There is considerable energy or 'error wisdom' (Reason, 2004) among front-line staff that we may fail to capitalise on.

The vignette highlights that what is needed is not purely clinical, technical and bureaucratic expertise, or expert-based knowledge, but also interpersonal, social, and organisational expertise. Indeed, this point was made some years ago in the *To Err is Human* report (US Institute of Medicine, 1999). Its view was that the general lack of intelligent organisation of clinical processes undermines what medicine can do at a technical level. In its view, doing medicine now is like 'manufacturing micro-processors in a vacuum tube factory':

> [A]ttempts to deliver today's technologies with today's medical production capabilities are the medical equivalent of manufacturing microprocessors in a vacuum tube factory . . . it will be even less able to carry the weight of tomorrow's technologies and an aging population, raising the spectre of even more variability in quality, more errors, less responsiveness, and greater costs associated with waste and poor quality. (US Institute of Medicine, 1999: 30)

It is for this reason too that commentators have begun to raise questions about patient safety and quality of care research methods and approaches. These questions ask why these methods and approaches privilege the technical, scientific and bureaucratic dimensions of care (approached through conventional medical-scientific methods) at the expense of the interpersonal, social and organisational dimensions of care (Leape *et al.*, 2002; Shojania *et al.*, 2001). Interestingly too, funding agencies in the industrialised world have begun to target studies that complement epidemiological-statistical evidence with research that captures the complexities of *in situ* experience.

All this shows that there is growing interest in methods and approaches that operate with narrative, visuals, discourse and ethnography. But these also have a draw-back: they are less amenable to cross-comparison and aggregation. This is so for two reasons: (1) their proximity to *in situ* complexity and (2) their own complex make-up.

Being close to *in situ* complexity does not just introduce 'noise'; it also reveals contradictions, paradoxes, and changeable answers. Close up, social and organisational phenomena are rarely simply black and white, and appear more likely in different shades of all sorts of colours. Video data, for example, are very rich and therefore time-consuming to produce and difficult to analyse (Pink, 2001). Not surprisingly, visual footage has predominantly been used for surveillance and assessment purposes. Video footage has enabled researchers and assessors to ascertain staff compliance with behavioural protocols and pedagogic prescriptions (e.g. Michaelson and Levi, 1997). While these uses are important, little use is in fact made of the handle on complexity that such methods and approaches make possible.

As the next chapter explains, quality and safety thinking has tended towards favouring simple answers, certainty, truth and generalisable expert knowledge. This thinking is accompanied by a fear that as soon as we leave room for contradiction, paradox and dynamics, we enter the domain of chaos, non-knowledge, subjective opinions and anti-order. Yet, for those who live the situations that these research methods and approaches seek to represent, contradiction, paradox and changeability (dynamics) are the order of the day.

For example, staff in the ICU know that they have to juggle information and intuition, they constantly have to hedge their bets, and continuously monitor both patients' situations and the unit's organisational dimensions, including staffing, beds and other specialties' interests and concerns (Carroll, 2009). Practitioners know that their care plans and treatment solutions are most likely temporary. In this environment, certainty comes at a premium.

Therefore, instead of acting purely on the strength of truths and certainties, staff in such units practise *adaptive behaviour* (Carroll, 2009): they structure what they know about medical science, clinical practice, organisational dynamics, staff constraints and individual patients into a workable present, a present that enables them 'to go on' (cf. Beckett, 1953; Wittgenstein, 1953). This interweaving of medical, clinical, organisational, staff and patient resources becomes the basis of clinicians' ability to act.

Knowing about the biophysiological significance of the patient's haemoglobin, the effect of relevant drugs, the availability of theatre and theatre staff, and the patient's condition in the here and now, clinicians have an array of means for establishing and intervening into how disease unfolds. Put together, these resources enable clinicians to maintain a degree of control, even when faced with multiple unpredictables. These resources provide opportunities for action and intervention. But all action is contingent on others' support, confirmation and continuation. Put differently, the continuity of the work depends on people acting as a team, as a collectivity. For this reason we will finish this chapter with a closer look at how people achieve and enact teamness, or collectivity.

The role of front-line intelligence in group collectivity

Enquiries into on-the-spot reparation of error-prone developments show that the way a team communicates and acts as a *collectivity* is critical to making work safe (Gherardi and Nicolini, 2002; Weick and Roberts, 1993). Effective teams manage risk and impending failure through interactive support, heedfulness and mindful communication. Central to these phenomena is *affect* as a medium via which information is relayed. Affect here refers to a sensibility that operates alongside, or behind, language. As it mobilises glances, gestures, facial expressions and other bodily resources, affect travels at high speed (Thrift, 2008) – a supervisor can spot in a split second whether a trainee is coping or not; a mother can sense within moments whether her disabled daughter will be safe in a particular care environment.

Applied to team work, affect operates in the form of ongoing mutual checking of activities and their consequences, sharing of tasks and renegotiating of knowledge and plans. In short, affect effects a type of *intervision* among actors (Dekker, 2005). It is that which enables team members in difficult situations to manage irregularities, uncertainties and problems (Iedema, *et al.*, 2010). The focus on video in the present book can now be explained as follows: video highlights and reveals relationships in their affective aspect.

This book's focus is therefore complementary to existing health care improvement, patient safety and health policy literatures, where safety is seen to be inherent in the team's culture, its leadership, in its adherence to evidence-based guidelines and rule-based practices. We now have a plethora of evidence-based guidelines (e.g. the Cochrane library), as well as research pointing to the limited 'compliance' of front-line staff with those guidelines (Mangione-Smith, *et al.*, 2007; McGlynn, *et al.*, 2003). There is research into what both error-averse culture and moral leadership look like 'on the ground' (McDonald *et al.*, 2010). In contrast, the organisational literature talks about the critical importance of affective conducts referred to in the previous paragraph: staff's mutual 'heedfulness' (Weick and Roberts, 1993), teams' 'mindfulness' (Weick, 2004), and practitioners' 'error wisdom' (Reason, 2004). The task now is to explain what characterises these affective conducts, and how they can be learned and shared.

Outside of health, there is quite a body of literature that delves deeply into team-based intelligence, where intelligence refers to the manifestation of positive affect. Of particular interest here is how teams manage the seemingly effortless distribution of knowledge and awareness across team members. These phenomena have also been described with terms such as 'collective competence' (Boreham, 2004) and 'distributed cognition' (Hutchins, 1995).

Central to these notions is the creation, by teams, of 'zones of collaborative attention' (Gherardi, 2007) and 'zones of legitimate peripheral participation' (Lave and Wenger, 1990). These zones are spaces and practices where novices can safely explore and begin to adopt the conducts of their superiors and of their profession's experts. They do so knowing they will be supportively supervised.

Gherardi's work in particular is important for showing that safety is inscribed not just into safe technologies and evidence-based rules, and not just into individuals' cognitive capacity. Instead, her work highlights how safety emerges from how teams practise, communicate and relate. Her studies are important for showing how individual team members' knowledge is rarely complete and exhaustive. The teams she describes need to have dialogue to put relevant knowledge and decisions together 'on the spot' to suit specific circumstances and challenges.

In health, the focus on *in situ* team processes has begun to strengthen over the last few years. We now have detailed descriptions of specialist team practices (Pope *et al.*, 2007; Smith *et al.*, 2003), team communication (Espin *et al.*, 2006; Lingard, *et al.*, 2005), team resilience (Wears *et al.*, 2008), and teams as micro-systems (Mohr, *et al.*, 2004). This work is beginning to open up the black box of frontline clinicians handle *in situ* clinical complexity. This work is critical therefore to enabling us to make informed judgements about those aspects of clinical complexity that are unlikely to ever be designed out (requiring creativity), and those which are in need of being redesigned (allowing prefiguration).

However, as argued earlier, designing work processes in the context of clinical complexity cannot just rely on producing abstract knowledge about these processes, putting rules in place for what should happen, and then telling front-line staff to 'go and do it'. What is needed is the development of a method for enhancing team members' confidence about how to interpret and then deploy such abstract resources, and thereby strengthen their own safety capacity. They are the people who face and live complexity, and they are therefore the ones who need to work together on containing it. They are the people who need to shift gears from a largely tacit collective competence into a more articulate distributed intelligence.

Of course, knowledge, rules and forcing functions are critical for many aspects of care, and they relieve front-line staff of having to be vigilant across too many work domains at once. However, we know that the complexity of clinical processes will only increase. There will be more staff migration, multi-morbidity, technologisation, socio-cultural 'churn', public expectation to have input into one's own care, involvement of patients and families in discussions about clinical incidents, and so forth, and so on. This means that clinical staff need to be provided with skills to handle complexity as much as their work needs to be made simpler.

In the next chapter, we enquire into the kinds of research that we have deployed to serve the quest of strengthening practitioners' safety capacity. We suggest that practical complexity may warrant being tackled using complex approaches; that is, approaches that set less store by being rigorous and inflexible than by being robust and flexible in the tracing and taming of practical complexity.

3

Does the complexity of care call for 'research complexity'?

Introduction

In the previous two chapters we stressed the increasing significance for frontline clinicians to be able to handle complex processes. We also listed the various reasons that explain why health care is becoming more and more complex. The argument we began to develop in the opening chapters is that too much emphasis has been placed on structuring health care to ensure it is safe, simple and evidence-based. Doing so is important, but it is not the full story.

Our concern with structure, standards, evidence and systems has turned us away from complexity, away from how day-to-day care unfolds. This has led us to overlook what happens *in situ*, dismissing its complexity as arbitrary to the bigger aim of rendering care safe. In doing this, we may have lost sight of the concerns of frontline professionals, because they work and live amidst complexity.

We accept that what happens in the here and now is defining of the safety and the quality of care provided, yet in our effort to further safety we wield abstractions (notwithstanding the powerful insights yielded by resources such as statistical process control) and generalisations (prescriptions about how to conduct handovers or theatre checks). It seems that in trying to help out frontline professionals, we privilege what we are comfortable with researching rather than confronting that which they find most challenging: the complexity of everyday work.

If we avoid confronting how complexity manifests *in situ*, we miss the opportunity to take account of how care is actually provided. We will put this more strongly: by not rendering *in situ* complexity focal we continue to take existing ways of providing care for granted. If we avoid the full complexity of *in situ* care provision, we disconnect our safety efforts from what practitioners do and say. Under such circumstances, we may satisfy ourselves that we have a blood transfusion guideline or a medical emergency team ('MET') system. However, we will never know how the guideline or the MET system is realised in our own service – how it works. We will not know how local opinions, conducts and constraints fill the 'gaps in reasoning' (Steinberg and Luce, 2005) that typify the guideline or system.

Not considering the *in situ* progress of care further means that we have not bothered to ask a number of critical questions. Can it be that engaging with *in situ* complexity offers important insights for how to make care safer? Since they are closest to it, should front-line practitioners and patients be involved in sharing and developing insights about safety? Would their involvement mean that we need new and different ways of accounting for how care is provided, what safety means, how safety comes about, and how clinical outcomes are framed?

In this book, our emphasis is on what front-line clinicians (and patients) do from moment to moment, taking account of the full complexity of *in situ* work. We emphasise that this is an important perspective. When we describe the specifics of how the clinical work unfolds (using ethnography and narrative-based methods) we do more than fill in details, or reveal the subjective and arbitrary aspects of what people do and say. On the contrary, we begin to come to terms with the complexity of *in situ* care work. As complexity is at the heart of the day-to-day reality of clinical practice we will devote this third chapter to exploring in greater detail how we can account for that complexity.

Complexity is a term that enables us to refer to an event without presuming that it has only one particular kind of cause, logic, interpretation or significance. Complex events embody many different phenomena, and they mean many different things for different people. Therefore, such events do not simply and linearly predetermine what will happen next. To act amidst complex events and to study such events means that we need to adopt 'complexity thinking' (Carroll, 2009) and 'complexity talking' (Iedema, 2011).

What are 'complexity thinking' and 'complexity talking'? We will answer these questions in the sections that follow. We start with a short historical overview of the genesis of complexity theory in science (*see* next section, 'Research as empowerment: a short historical overview of scientific development'). Central here is how science (such as physics and chemistry) underwent a major shift in theoretical and methodological thinking, from Cartesian-Newtonian principles towards complexity thinking (Dekker, 2011). We discuss how science was forced to articulate its own assumptions, perspectives and constraints – in short, its own complexity. Significantly, and perhaps paradoxically, this articulation set the scene for science's capacity to confront and account for ('talk about') complex phenomena.

Following on from that, we demonstrate the relevance of this new way of thinking to complex social and organisational phenomena, of which clinical work is a prime example (*see* 'Complexity thinking and health care research', p. 50). The fact that clinical work is deeply complex, we will argue, explains the need for both formal procedures *and* at-work learning. This learning presupposes that frontline professionals can talk about the complexities they experience. Last, we turn our attention to the relationship between researching complex kinds of work, including 'doing safety', and *exnovation* (*see* 'The complexity of safety improvement research', p. 56). This prepares us for the fourth chapter of this book, which will be devoted to elaborating the principles and practice of exnovation using video-reflexive ethnography.

Research as empowerment: a short historical overview of scientific development

Research, as the term suggests, is an activity anchored in 'seeking again'. This activity of 'seeking again' is done purposefully: to re-present or make explicit what is found. Making things, experiences and events explicit in language is central to being human. For the German philosopher Sloterdijk, making phenomena explicit ('explicitation') is the civilising act par excellence:

> Here becomes manifest again the movement towards explicitation of which we know that it drives and guides civilisations to portray themselves to and for themselves. Explicitation breaks open what has remained confused in closedness and adds new discoveries and inventions to those already brought into existence. (Sloterdijk, 2009)[7]

In making matters explicit, research opens them up to becoming functional in ways they were not before. On the other hand, Bruno Latour, a well-known

---

7   Our translation. The original German reads: 'Hier zeigt sich erneut die explizitmachende Bewegung, von der wir wissen, daß sie den Weg der Zivilisation zur kognitiven Selbstdarstellung antriebt und begleitet. Explikation bricht das in konfuser Erschlossenheit Vorgefundene auf und fügt dem Aggregat des schon Entdeckten weitere Entdeckungen hinzu. Dabei verschieben sich die Grenzen zwischen dem Üblichen und dem Üngewöhnlichen . . .' (Sloterdijk, 2009: 298)

anthropologist of science, refers to research as an activity that renders phenomena *portable* (Latour, 1986).[8] Being rendered portable means that a phenomenon can now be addressed, manipulated and re-represented away from where it exists. This enables people to act on it 'from a distance'.

Let's take the example of a health service. It could be considered from the perspective of how many people make use of it; what its general outcomes are; how much it costs on a yearly basis; and how many full-time, part-time and casual staff it employs. Here, research enables us to create a perspective on health care processes and expenditures that might otherwise remain unremarked and therefore unremarkable. Now that we have conceptualised processes and expenditures as means for 'framing' the care provided by that service, we can begin to act on these dimensions through improvement initiatives, or resource redistributions. Here, action has become possible 'from a distance' thanks to specialised forms of language used by actors far removed from the day-to-day work: managers, health department officials, accreditation surveyors, and so forth.

As a form of 'explicitation', research is deeply inscribed into the human psyche. This is because humankind, as 'the symbolic species' (Deacon, 1997), re-presents aspects of its own existence to gain access to them, and control over them. The ability to create new symbolic perspectives on phenomena has even played a central role in human evolution (Edelman, 1992). For Edelman and Deacon, the mainstay of human evolution was and is ongoing symbolisation and re-presentation of aspects of existence, or what Sloterdijk calls explicitation.

This re-presentational momentum gained extra intensity in the seventeenth century during the so-called Age of Enlightenment. The Enlightenment prioritised 'reason' as the primary source of legitimacy and authority. What 'reason' came down to in reality is this: the Enlightenment was a period of intense specialisation targeting the re-presentation of natural phenomena such that humans could more easily manipulate them (Porter, 2001). An apple falling to the ground is not just 'the way things are'; it represents a law of nature – gravity. This law can now be applied to a whole range of objects. Gravity provides a symbolic abstraction that connects how objects behave in general.

Similarly, people getting sick is not just 'what happens (to individuals)': it is now re-presented as a complex bio-physiological process involving lesions whose nature and growth can be linked to classes of diseases occurring in humans generally, and for which we can design treatments with varying levels of effectiveness

---

8   Latour uses the term 'immutable mobile' to refer to the outcome of this process of re-presentation of phenomena (Latour, 1986).

(Foucault, 1973). For all these reasons, research can empower humans, because it enables them to change their circumstances. Research extends the scope of human agency into domains where, previously, limited action was possible, effective or useful. Language, or 'discourse', plays a central role here: through ongoing specialisation, discourse frames 'the real' in increasingly distinctive and explicit terms.

This paradigm of 'explicitation', the one that has driven and is still driving research, is also one of objectification. This means turning complex physical, bio-physiological and social phenomena into carefully delimited objects. Water falling from the sky comes to be known as 'precipitation'. It is this project of delimiting and naming phenomena that enables science to conduct its research business (Martin, 1993). Phenomena are credited with boundaries, and this framing makes them manipulable. Or at least, we can start asking questions about how they can be made manipulable.

The discovery of insulin is a good example of this. It started in 1896 with Langerhans discovering previously unnoticed clumps of tissue in the pancreas, which subsequently became known as 'the islets of Langerhans'. Research into their function found a link with diabetes when dogs deprived of their pancreas started to produce overly sweet urine. The islets became the focus of much research activity all over the world. This was until, in the 1920s in Canada, islet extracts were shown to regulate blood sugar levels (Bliss, 2011). The identification, or *making explicit*, of pancreatic tissue islets made possible focused research activity into digestive bodily processes and functions, producing one of the most profound discoveries of the twentieth century: insulin.

Of course, science relies on a wealth of techniques and technologies (Latour and Woolgar, 1979). But scientific practice is unthinkable without the ongoing *discursive* classification and categorisation of phenomena. Science will classify and categorise all sorts of phenomena, many of which may have appeared initially to be too ephemeral (e.g. the weather) or too complex (e.g. social phenomena) to afford coherent descriptions. Classification and categorisation enable the scientist to freeze-frame phenomena of interest, and this enables them to experiment with them and investigate their relationships (Bowker and Star, 1999).

How we name or 'represent' things (making 'present again' by making explicit) thus plays a prominent role in our creation of knowledge about the world. Representation makes such things and our knowledge about them portable: we can point to them and observe across settings and contexts. This strategy, in turn, means we are able to enhance the way we act on and in the world. Put more formally, we extend the reach of our human agency by reframing, innovating, and technologising the ways in which we frame and act on the world around us (Rossi-Landi, 1975). The more phenomena become objectified, the more they become amenable to manipulation.

The advantages of this paradigm of objectification are well known. Galileo, Newton and Einstein were great luminaries because they were able to re-present phenomena that everyone else had accepted to be just the way they were. These scientists reframed our worlds in far-reaching ways, with far-reaching conse-quences for how we now live our lives. Yet, and perhaps surprisingly in light of these achievements, the paradigm of thought that inspired so much insight, power and progress started to come up against its own limits. Let us outline a number of reasons for this dilemma.

First, the insights produced by quantum theory in the early twentieth century led physicists to conclude that their methods of observation were not neutral and innocent. That is, their procedures were no longer seen to be merely transparent means to visualising what was 'out there'. Instead, every method and technique to observe reality was found to be a particular framing of this reality. This realisation had all sorts of consequences for how reality was seen and understood. Scientific methods were realised to carry a host of assumptions about the reality they were supposed to 'objectively' analyse and define.

Scientists started to realise that there was no way out: with every method of observation a host of assumptions and values slipped into scientific observations and measurements. Observation and measurement could no longer be seen to be value-free, produced by scientists adopting a 'view from nowhere' (Nagel, 1989). They realised that scientific observation, instead of mirroring what is 'out there', is predisposed and even determined by the methods and instruments it mobilises to do its work (Prigogine and Stengers, 1984).

This made scientists realise that instead of observing and measuring 'the real', they were in fact party to how the real was made observable and measurable. This realisation opened up a whole new way of understanding whose principal point of departure was now *complexity* and *complexity thinking* (Prigogine and Stengers, 1984).

Complexity thinking was particularly evident in the work of early twentieth-century physicists such as Bohr and Heisenberg. They began to explore the philosophical implications inherent in what they were doing as scientists. For them, science could no longer be understood as an enterprise that provides a more and more detailed view of 'the real', filling in more and more gaps in knowl-edge until we fully understand the workings of reality (Barad, 1998, 2003). By applying the standards of investigative openness and consistency to scientific practices and methods, they laid bare the compromises they saw as inseparable from scientific progress (Babich *et al.*, 1995). With this, and while science continued to intensify its programme of extending the reach and power of human agency, scientists could no longer regard doing science as simply laying bare 'the real' (Barad, 2003).

Demonstrating people's mounting concern about these questions, the twentieth century produced a burgeoning philosophy of science (Harré, 1972; Kuhn, 1962; Prigogine, 1996) as well as intense debates and radical revisions (Feyerabend, 1975). Choosing a method and an approach now inevitably means settling for particular assumptions and values. This is done in the knowledge that these assumptions and values are likely to be contestable, if not already contested. There is thus a curious paradox that shadows twentieth-century science. Recent science may have enabled us to radically extend our agency into the world and into space, assisting in the technologisation of practices, transportation, migration, social and institutional change, and so forth. However, none of these developments would have come about without science turning its own lens on itself.

By opening itself up to investigation and by investigating itself, science has foregrounded the assumptions, values and investments that drive and sustain it. In doing so, science revealed that it could no longer be understood as a neutral means to representing and capturing 'the real'. Instead, it came to be understood as a complex endeavour that links a diversity of efforts, interests and investments. It is an endeavour that operates with multivariate perspectives, partial benefits, contestable outcomes and ethical implications. In admitting these things, science situates itself amidst the domain of complexity, and engages in what Montuori terms 'complexity thinking' (Montuori, 2003).

Complexity thinking

What are the implications of the above account for how we study health care? One important implication affects the status we accord to our research approaches. It is naïve to continue to pretend that some research approaches have privileged access to truth, and that some are better at articulating cause–effect relationships. Both observational studies and large-scale studies have limitations, albeit different ones. Both produce 'truths' of specific kinds. Both draw their own conclusions, with observational studies generally highlighting the overdetermined nature of actions and events, and large-scale studies emphasising simplified causal correlations between phenomena. Depending on the time, place and use to which they are put, both can be effective, or harmful, in promoting their findings and conclusions.

Ultimately, what is critical is that we learn from these different kinds of studies without being so naïve as to assume that some kinds are more capable of revealing 'the truth' than others. Someone who writes about these issues, Sidney Dekker, regards cause–effect investigations as integral to doing investigations into things that went wrong, but he dismisses the idea that we can come to an absolute determination of cause–effect relationships (Dekker, 2005). Claiming that any particular approach is capable of determining what caused particular events is propaganda, he suggests. Such claims lapse into what he terms 'Cartesian-Newtonian thinking' – thinking that ignores developments in the very sciences (physics, philosophy) that spawned and then questioned such thinking (Dekker, 2011). Cartesian-Newtonian thinking maintains that we can adopt a 'view from nowhere', and that we can make absolute pronouncements about 'the real'. For Dekker, the idea that we can make such pronouncements is naïve.

Dekker explains that, in our complex world, we need a multiplicity of approaches and answers to cope with the uncertainty that permeates everyday practice and decision-making. In health care, uncertainty is pervasive. Medical diagnoses are found to be frequently (in 50% of cases) confounded by unexplainable symptoms (Nimnuan *et al.*, 2001) and around 80% of what doctors do is not evidence-based (Jorm, 2012). In negotiations about what to do about a disease, patients' own preferences and organisational resource constraints are factors that add further uncertainty. All this means that the practice of medicine is complex, and that to understand how this practice unfolds we need methods other than ones that simplify 'the real' down to its most basic and sterile causal chains. In this context, and thanks to the methods and approaches it mobilises, social research is capable of tackling such complexity. Indeed, the pervasive complexity in health care renders social research *critical and central* to what health care is and does.

The position of research in social life generally has shifted from a few peculiar interests of a handful of scientists, to a pervasive activity by numerous researchers who explore a bewildering array of aspects of living (Taylor, 1985). We research everything from people's spending patterns, children's eating habits, patients' journeys through a service, to clinicians' working practices and administrators' accounting processes. Few spheres of life remain unresearched. While much research is promoted as being necessary 'to fill a knowledge gap', the irony is that the more we come or assume to know about the world, the more complexity comes to the fore, every time opening up new panoramas of existence that are yet to be named, described and understood. The more we name, describe and (claim to) understand, the greater the pressure to name, describe and understand 'new' phenomena. Every discovery produces more complexity. The further we reach into the universe, the more planets and galaxies come into view, and the more we sense its potential infinity.

All this means that the real is not a finite territory to be mapped out (like the earth), but a perspective-dependent universe that keeps on expanding away from us as we move into it and through it. The term 'fractal' was introduced to characterise this latter experience: what we see, or assume to see, extends away from us in never-ending and self-resembling patterns, or fractals. It has also been hypothesised that the reason we find things arranged in fractals is that they are an expression of our way of seeing, defined and shaped by human perception. The other thing we know about fractals is that they may make things appear to be quite structured, but that such arrangements or structures can at any time be disturbed and knocked apart. Complexity is omnipresent.

Perhaps because we have trained ourselves to see it, complexity is now accepted to be omnipresent. Complexity is now taken to be so pervasive, and affect existing arrangements and structures to such an extent that we have begun to talk about 'the end of certainty' (Prigogine, 1996).

Prigogine, the Nobel Laureate who coined the phrase 'the end of certainty', is a physicist who (with Isabelle Stengers) formalised scientists' growing sense of complexity into 'complexity theory' (Prigogine and Stengers, 1984). Complexity theory acknowledges that 'the real' is not some stable entity answering to universal laws. Instead 'the real' is a complex dynamic that answers to 'strange attractors'. Strange attractors are shifting and at times radically perturbed patterns that can at any time re-pattern in completely different ways. This process is labelled 'dynamic complexity'. Dynamic complexity refers to a constantly changing field of forces constituting and affected by natural phenomena and human activities. Importantly, then, the term complexity here points to the *changeable* nature of existence, and the *multifactorial* nature of the causes of those changes. The term complexity further invokes the *unpredictability* of our future, not least because of the *reflexive* impact of humans making sense of and thereby further perturbing the dynamics in which they are implicated, rather than accepting and living them blindly (Prigogine, 1996).

Understandably too, and this is why we explained the genesis of complexity theory, our approaches to doing science are multiplying. Science is no longer the discrete domain it used to be, locked away in stable disciplines and in carefully sealed labs pursuing specialisation in order to 'fill gaps in knowledge'. On the contrary, science is increasingly multidisciplinary, with scientists working across knowledge boundaries within scientific fields as well as across the disciplinary boundaries that used to separate types of science, or 'hard' science from social science, art and the humanities.

Science is also increasingly being conducted outside of labs in its attempt to understand complexity unaffected by artificial limiting conditions. Indeed, boundary-spanning is as common and true in science as it is in contemporary social research. Here, crossover areas like 'sci-art' are increasingly common and varied, blending practices and insights from very different fields and disciplines.

Complexity thinking and health care research

Boundary-spanning is also occurring in the field of patient safety, where debates are now in full swing about methodology, the status of findings and the importance of theory to locate our 'view from somewhere' (Berwick, 2008; Grol *et al.*, 2008; Lohr, 2007; Shojania and Grimshaw, 2005). These debates take place against a background of classic 'hierarchy of evidence' thinking. In relative ignorance of the developments in science described earlier, the 'hierarchy of evidence' principle posits that the grander the scale of the research approach and procedure, the more valid and reliable the findings.

Calling these principles into doubt, recent debates in health and safety research are now acknowledging we need to engage with the problem of how to approach and intervene in health care complexity. These debates are beginning to clarify that to understand complexity we need more fine-grained approaches (Berwick, 2007). The problem that is becoming evident is that the process of applying generalised knowledge and procedural rules to specific actions and events is not straightforward, and perhaps not even the right way to think about change, improvement and reform.

In the previous chapter we addressed the complex nature of health care work. There, we discussed events that are untypical, that are interpreted differently, and that may entrain all kinds of unpredictabilities. We acknowledged that in many situations clinicians will be able to fall back on skills, expertise and strict routines (Vincent, 2006). However, we also concluded that safety in contemporary health care is increasingly contingent on rapid turnarounds and creative solutions tailored to cope with the constantly shifting configuration of people, resources, skills, problems and needs.

What we need to ask now is: what is needed for those front-line practitioners to feel comfortable acting amidst complexity? The question that follows on from this one is: what kind of research engages with the problems and challenges that front-line practitioners encounter in their everyday work, and how can it benefit those at the front line?

To answer these questions, let us first explore in greater detail what confounds practitioners. First, there are the practical consequences of their constantly expanding and specialising professional skill set and expert knowledge. The emphasis on furthering the scientific dimensions of medicine at the expense of its organisational and communicative dimensions means that, as mentioned in Chapter 2, doing medicine nowadays is like 'manufacturing microprocessors in a vacuum tube factory':

> [A]ttempts to deliver today's technologies with today's medical production capabilities are the medical equivalent of manufacturing microprocessors in a vacuum tube factory . . . it will be even less able to carry the weight of tomorrow's technologies and an aging population, raising the spectre of even more variability in quality, more errors, less responsiveness, and greater costs associated with waste and poor quality. (US Institute of Medicine, 1999: 30)

Our research lens tends to be trained on the formal science of medicine and on the bureaucratisation of care provision (Harrison *et al.*, 2002) rather than the everyday enactment of care. We are thereby leaving the problem of how to enact care entirely to front-line clinicians and patients. Metaphorically speaking, it is they who are burdened with 'manufacturing microprocessors in a vacuum tube factory'. Front-line practitioners are the ones expected to forge a bridge from increasingly invasive curative techniques and bureaucratic directives, to the mundane decisions about what these techniques and directives mean for individual patients' care trajectories.

In forging that bridge, they traverse a terrain swarming with uncertainties. Patients presenting with unclear symptoms lead to diagnostic uncertainty: is the patient suffering from cholecystitis, pneumonia, or both? Unless they have a collaborative approach to addressing and resolving such questions, considerable tension can divide teams until test results offer some clarity. As these deliberations unfold, patients can expect to see up to 300 different clinicians during a single week in hospital (Degeling *et al.*, 2001), and be asked questions by up to 40 emergency department staff over a 4-hour period in the emergency department (Manidis and Scheeres, 2012). When we consider care as it unfolds, we become aware of the considerable uncertainty that permeates it.

This uncertainty is exacerbated by clinician practitioners' moving from role to role through the care system, and by junior doctors rotating through departments, in addition to services' increasing reliance on 'casual' agency nursing and medical locum staff. Uncertainty also springs from ongoing technologisation in the domains of information and communications technologies, diagnostic technologies and pharmaceutical developments. What adds to this 'technological swirl' is the rapid turnover and constant updating of these technologies. As if this were not enough, the frequent absence of organisation- and specialty-wide agreements about how to provide specific medical-surgical treatments manifests in arbitrary variations in the ways in which treatments and care are structured.

Then there is the changing relationship between clinicians and patients. Here, there is much interpersonal uncertainty. Patients expect their care to be increasingly communication-based: they are to be consulted extensively about procedures. Communication intensifies even more when care goes wrong, with clinicians and services having to explain what happened (Iedema *et al.*, 2011).

Overall, pressure on how and what clinicians communicate is growing because of the rising number of stakeholders in health. Indeed, contemporary health care is an increasingly *'crowded space'* (Little, 1994). Not just multiple health care professionals, but also bioethicists, consumer representatives, health care complaints commissioners, 'clinical excellence commissions' and 'safety and quality' staff, and 'health care commissions' made up of policymakers are assuming a look at and a say in what clinicians do for and with patients. Each of these players demands different kinds of communicative attention, whether in the form of 'informed consent', clinical outcome statistics, resource utilisation reports, or patient satisfaction survey data. This multiplication of discourses about health care problematises rather than simplifies the question about how to represent particular aspects of care. For example, how do we talk about an unexpected outcome in care such as an overdose of insulin leading to an ICU admission? Is it a systems' failure, an individual's error, or the result of a complex chain of actions and events? Together, uncertainties such as these render *in situ* care highly complex.

Back in the 1960s, commentators had already claimed that 'no one knows what the hospital "is" on any given day unless he [*sic*] has a comprehensive grasp of what combination of rules and policies, along with agreements, understandings, pacts, contracts, and other working arrangements, currently obtains' (Strauss *et al.*, 1963: 164). By implication, such grasp was then near enough impossible. Now, such grasp is unthinkable, both for experienced clinicians who devote themselves to particular specialties or units and for junior clinicians for whom 'knowing what the hospital is' remains elusive despite the many hours they spend in the service, and their rotation through various departments and specialties.

Now, how do these considerations impact on questions about how we study and enhance patient safety? We will answer this question by delving further into how practitioners accomplish safety, *in situ*.

Practitioners frequently have to navigate through multiple constraints, and in doing so they devise answers, solutions and ways forward from what comes to hand. This process – fashioning solutions from what comes to hand – is essentially a creative performance. It involves practitioners collectively and creatively executing their tasks. In doing so, they co-enact (to greater or lesser extent) what can be referred to as their 'collective competence' (Boreham, 2004).

Collective competence refers to what collectives of people can do thanks to belonging to the group, and members of the group complementing each other's knowledge and action. The following vignette demonstrates this principle: clinicians negotiate a variety of demands and constraints simultaneously *in situ*, in the 'liminal' space of the corridor (the term 'liminal' captures the idea of something being in the margins). Here, we see a doctor and a social worker negotiating how to tie on an infection control gown (Extract 3.1). This event happened a couple of days before the encounter described in Chapter 2 (Extract 2.1). In Chapter 2, we saw how the doctor and the nurse ran into the occupational therapist and began discussing an intensive care unit patient's mattress. Interrupting the discussion, the nurse advised the occupational therapist that she should tie her gown round her back. The doctor then confessed that he 'can't do the back tie'. This comment shows that he remembers the importance of tying his gown round his back from the earlier event that is portrayed here in Vignette 3.1.

This vignette reveals how the doctor advises the social worker that he should put on a gown. Then, the ward nurse corrects both the doctor and the social worker: their gown should be tied round their back, not their front.

The significance of this sequence lies in the fact that it shows these clinicians as sharing two crucial resources: (1) they are attentive to each other's actions and (2) they have a language for communicating about each other's (inappropriate) actions. Safety, in this apparently mundane encounter, emerges not just from what individuals know, nor just from individuals following strict procedures, but from team members communicating with each other in *ad hoc* ways about matters that arise in the course of ongoing action. Knowledge and procedures are in play, but these are ultimately enabled and rendered functional as a result of the attentive and communicative work done *in situ* by the members of the team.

Vignette 3.1

Corridor sequence outside procedures room: doctor commences gowning, social worker enters procedures room without gown or gloves.

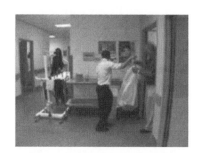

Doctor: Do you want a gown, Don [social worker]?

Social worker comes back, doctor hands social worker gown.

Social worker: Oh, thanks.

Doctor gets gown for himself.

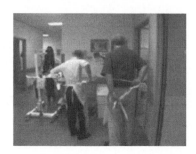

Doctor and social worker gown up.

Doctor walks up corridor tying apron around the front. Sticks head in consult room A and walks out again.

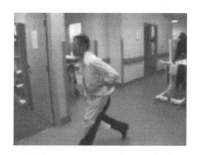

[...]

Doctor walks back towards procedures room, nurse exits consult room A and follows.

Nurse: Um, Kim [*doctor turns, nurse indicates apron*], don't tie it round the front.[9]
Doctor: Uh, OK, sorry.

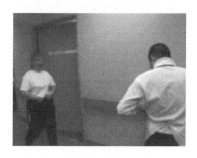

Doctor re-ties apron at the back.

---

9   Tying the gown around the front creates the risk of the apron strings making contact with infected bodies and thereby infecting the clinician's hands upon untying the apron.

There are two other things to be learned from this vignette. First, the sequence shows that adequate knowledge of procedures is likely to be *distributed* across team members (Hutchins, 1995; Hutchins and Klausen, 1998). Thus, the doctor advised the social worker about the importance of putting on the gown and gloves; the nurse advised both on the importance of tying the gown round their back. This is critical because not one single person will be able to know (or have the time to advise others on) everything there is to know about the various safety aspects of the work (Kunda, 1992). Therefore, team members have to communicate about these matters as the work unfolds, about what is important to know about the work, and about the multiple safeties that need to be performed as part of the work (namely, putting on a gown and gloves; tying the gown around the back). This non-formal process of knowledge sharing is central to enabling practitioners to do their work and do it safely, and it is critical to team members enhancing their and each other's skills (Eraut, 2004).

Second, and as a logical extension of this first point, the distribution of work-relevant knowledge depends on how, and how much, team members *communicate about* it. The more opportunity team members have to talk about facets of the work, the more chance there is that the knowledge distribution network will be enriched and remain up to speed. Equally, an active, dynamic knowledge distribution network is more likely to reinforce and enhance individuals' knowledge and capacities. As individuals they are also more likely to shift from a position of learner engaging in non-critical activity or 'peripheral participation' to that of expert engaging in a more central (to the practice) type of participation (Engeström, 2008). This learning, we contend, takes practitioners beyond their collective competence into a new space: the space of *distributed intelligence*.

We may witness collective competence in action when we walk into an emergency department (Boreham *et al.*, 2000). Clinicians may engage in highly skilful manoeuvres, many of which complement one another, but many of which may also be hugely dissonant (Manidis, 2013). For practitioners to address and intervene in the habituated dimensions of what they do and resolve those dissonances, they need to develop ways of subjecting their collective competence to reflexive deliberation (Iedema, 2011). Such deliberation may convert collective competence into shared learning. Shared learning is the basis of distributed intelligence.

On this view, care and safety cannot be reduced to people's personal or even their shared (tacit and explicit) knowledges and activities. Rather, doing safety is about clinicians co-producing new futures – a process that can be described using Ticineto-Clough's phrase 'futurising the present' (Ticineto-Clough, 2008). 'Futurising the present' refers to the constant assessment, scenario-building and forward projection of scenarios (Mitchell, 2009) in which actors engage to maximise their agency and effectiveness in practical situations. Because it is manifest in and as shared action, 'futurising' is observable and describable. Thinking back to the vignette seen above, the clinicians there think ahead about the consequences of not tying on a gown, and of not tying the gown correctly.

'Futurising the present' differs in an important way from collective competence. The latter imputes the existence of a weave of mutual attention and commitment, but it says nothing about clinicians' ability to intervene in their own and each other's competences. Futurising the present is different. It refers to professionals' ability and willingness to scrutinise and reinvent their own and each other's conduct. To achieve this, they need to be able to extrapolate from existing behaviours and activities, base scenarios on them that extend into the future, and evaluate the consequences were these scenarios to eventuate, all *in vacuo*. Framed in this way, futurising produces a meta-perspective.

For the behaviours at issue here to become visible, we need to mobilise new approaches and new methods. These approaches and methods are unusual in that they key in to the complexities and dynamics of mundane, everyday practice.

The complexity of safety improvement research

The uncertainty affecting care, the diversification of practices and the growing multitude of stakeholders point to a need for research approaches that can accommodate the dynamic complexity of these behaviours on the part of front-line clinicians. Such approaches must recognise that the application of appropriate rules and expert knowledge to care are but isolated aspects of what practitioners do *in situ*. They recognise also that safety depends in an important way on how professionals work together: whether and how they create a shared intelligence for observing and addressing routines and practices. Such approaches recognise that such intelligence is dynamic, reflexive and emergent, and therefore contingent on ongoing dialogue.

To date, we have but limited insight into practitioners' safety-maintaining and safety-creating practices (Mesman, forthcoming). Human factors researchers have begun to describe aspects of these processes using the concept of '*resilience*'. Over time, the term resilience was expanded to encompass both reactive behaviours compensating for problems, and proactive ones targeting learning from those problems (Hollnagel, 2006; Hollnagel *et al.*, 2006). Resilience research now distinguishes between 'safety¹', referring to research that attempts to eradicate errors and failures, and 'safety[2]', referring to research that is interested in ordinary, everyday performance (Hollnagel, 2012). Hollnagel dismisses safety[1] – trying to derive safety principles from the minority of incidents and accidents that perturb practice. He regards safety[2] (the focus on care that is not subject to incidents) as a far more productive way to understand safety.

While Hollnagel's view might seem to parallel the one presented in this book, his distinction between safety[1] and safety[2] sits uneasily with the views espoused here. This is because, for us, the opposition between 'faulty practice' and 'successful practice' is tenuous. It is based on a distinction that we find difficult to make. We regard the safety of practice not just as a continuous, ongoing accomplishment but also as an accomplishment that is both highly vulnerable and rarely perfect, but also mostly 'safe enough'.

Indeed, practice is never fully safe or fully unsafe. Rather, safety and unsafety permeate practice in unpredictable ways. A simple, standard procedure (to use Lillrank and Liukko's term introduced in Chapter 2) harbours the potential for veering into unsafe territory and complete failure. By the same token, a complex practice will manifest as a patchwork of 'safeties' and 'unsafeties'. There, the safety gradient of what practitioners do may depend on what trade-offs are made. Think back to the choice surgeons may need to make between the speed of using flexible reusable devices and the safety of sterile but inflexible throwaways (Rowley, 2011). Advantages and disadvantages attach to both devices, but some will be preferable in particular situations. In short, only in idealisations will practice manifest as a homogeneous, self-same collection of phenomena. When considered close-up, practice is more likely to manifest as a jumble of different, potentially unrelated and perhaps even incongruous things, actions and decisions.

To understand practice and safety, we need to account for the incongruities that connect things, actions and decisions. To date, there remains a dearth of research into how the problem of navigating and trading off 'safeties' and 'unsafeties' manifests for practitioners, how it can be recognised, and how it can be explained and conveyed to those who are as yet unreceptive to it. This also suggests that the means for engendering capacity among practitioners for dealing with such problems remains underspecified. We do not have a pedagogy (or rather, an 'andragogy') for learning from complexity, for acting amidst complexity, nor for reinventing practice that unfolds under complex conditions. We do not know how to prepare clinicians for *adaptive* practice, and we do not know how to enable them to deliberate about their adaptive responses.

One thing that is becoming increasingly evident in all this is that complexity demands *specification* rather than generalisation. When we specify what happened in specific situations, we become able to deal with some of their and other situations' complexities. Understanding specific circumstances and events pays off when similar circumstances and events arise later and elsewhere. This is how Greenhalgh and colleagues express this idea:

> The scholar who studies a painting of a tree by Cézanne and discusses with others its meaning and significance does not learn about merely this particular painting or the tree in it. Rather, he or she will also look with a more sophisticated eye at other Impressionist paintings and other trees. (Greenhalgh *et al.*, 2011: 545)

In pursuing the question 'what is going on here', we may not benefit much from vague generalisations. In contrast, specification inspires our sensitivity to and articulacy about complex phenomena. Specification may give us confidence to deal with the rapidly changing circumstances and scenarios in which we find ourselves, because we have encountered similarly complex situations before. Specification sensitises us to nuances, distinctions, subtle dynamics and intimate details. Moreover, specification provides us with a discourse for deliberating about and engaging with such details.

No doubt it is for that reason that the case study plays such a prominent role in 'case law' and in medicine (namely, the 'case report'), where sophisticated knowledge of details and fine-grained distinctions are important (Kennedy, 1979). Our interest in specificity takes us down the path of uniqueness, away from the main road of truth paved with abstract norms and general advice. Delving into the specificity of cases may prepare us for complex circumstances by strengthening our ability to recognise them.

Yet most research in health services and safety is based on the assumption that we can and must derive rules about causation. These laws are taken to be necessary for predicting the future and thereby enabling action: if we act according to the evidence, good outcomes will ensue. But this faith in absolute laws and causation is a form of Cartesian-Newtonian thinking (Dekker, 2011). Cartesian-Newtonian thinking manifests in the assumption that knowing the past and understanding its laws are both necessary and sufficient for predicting and defining future action.

However, this thinking erases from view the fact that practitioners need to self-organise in the face of *in situ* challenges, problems and opportunities. An example of such dynamic, self-organising and collaborative activity was seen earlier, where a clinical team assisted one another with raising their level of infection control. Self-organising may involve adapting a rule to suit a context (Ovretveit, 2011), but it may also go beyond that. It may require a 'bricolage' of rules, technologies, information, insights, knowledge and resources. Indeed, it may require a truly creative response that goes beyond existing rules and knowledge to suit resource constraints and circumvent impending risks.

This brings us to the following related point. Researching how work *ought* to be done, and assessing to what extent work done compares to how it ought to be done, may be easier than studying how practitioners bring safety into being in a dynamic and creative way. The former tasks measure action against clearly predefined parameters: the pathway, the guideline, the checklist, the benchmarked outcome. The latter maps how safety emerges from *in situ* communication, and this may include ad hoc comments, glances, gestures, cryptic utterances, opportunistic decisions, gut feelings and chance observations. This latter focus may also encompass staff chatting in tearooms or corridors about vexing problems, or their unease about aspects of their practice (Iedema *et al.*, 2010). This latter domain is the most complex to research, because it focuses on the most complex dimensions of safety. These dimensions include not just the adaptive, emergent processes of clinicians and patients 'doing safety' in the here and now, but also their unplanned deliberations about how to proceed, and their discussions about how to reshape established practice.

While several aspects of clinical work may be predictable and able to be made into procedures (Begun and Kaissi, 2004), many are also increasingly challenging for reasons already enumerated here: technologisation, staff turnover, resource constraints, public expectations, rising numbers of very elderly patients with chronic diseases and co-morbidities, policy reform, and so forth. To iterate some of the language used in Chapter 2, it may be that in this day and age fewer activities are standard and predictable, more are routine (requiring a degree of judgement), and even more are predominantly non-routine, requiring sophisticated kinds of judgement and decision-making (Lillrank and Liukko, 2004).

Research and improvement science need to address and account for this rising complexity and for the implications it has for practice. Approaches need to be devised and deployed that can tackle this complexity, particularly where it is most acute: at the front line where care is delivered to patients (Manidis and Scheeres, 2012). There, complexity manifests in people more frequently having to communicate with one another about more things. In that regard, work is becoming increasingly 'communication-intense' (Deetz, 1995). Communication acts as the medium with which we address and resolve complex tasks.

Researching how people achieve safety thus needs to involve making sense of how (and whether!) clinicians communicate with one another. This includes mapping and tracing information-sharing practices, but also observing *how* people engage with one another. Here questions such as these become important: Do people have opportunities for raising issues that matter to them? How do these opportunities play out for them? Do they play out as interruptions to critical routines, or are they welcomed? Are these opportunities planned to occur? In taking the opportunity to raise important issues, do people talk about the ways they act and communicate? That is, do they have a *meta-discourse* for how they communicate, about what, and when (Iedema *et al.*, 2009e)?

To establish whether these kinds of communication occur we need to stay close to them, follow them around, and map or trace the conversations they encounter and generate over time. This is not so that we will capture the totality of what they do, since that is per definition impossible as well as practically unnecessary. Rather, such research involves getting sufficiently close to what clinicians do and say to notice what we otherwise cannot see: the collective reasoning that informs what they do and how they do it. It is important to capture that reasoning because it is an indicator of their distributed intelligence. Defined thus, the research that is needed to understand 'doing safety' relies on proximity to *practice*.[10]

Proximity to practice is not merely for the benefit of researchers, such that they may discern how safety is done. It is also beneficial for clinicians themselves. Potentially motivated by researchers' attention on their *in situ* routines, clinicians may equally be inspired and enabled to gain insight into their own communication and actions. When clinicians become involved in explorations of this kind, they may become self-conscious. More often than not, however, they become excited about the possibility of understanding what they do from moment to moment. This may give them confidence to nurture awareness of their own communication and work practices. This, in turn, enables them to develop a *meta-discourse* for articulating how they relate and communicate with

---

10 The rising concern about diagnostic errors in recent times is interesting in this regard (e.g. Schiff *et al.*, 2009). In fact, diagnostic decisions are influenced by individual clinicians' expertise levels, clinicians' collective ways of working (clinicians working collaboratively or not), and their documentation practices. Where exactly the diagnostic moment is to be located remains unclear from the literature that addresses diagnostic errors, as if that is a non-issue. This moment's proximity to and dependence on available expertise, *in situ* practice and documentation routines should be evident. In acknowledging this however, we encounter some important questions: to what extent are diagnostic errors traceable to sub-standard inter- and intra-professional support, supervision, team-work, documentation, IT set-up? Where do we draw the boundary? And what does that say about the accuracy we wish to invest in identifying and classifying 'diagnostic errors'?

one another. Such meta-discourse means they can begin to play a critical reflexive role in how they work and communicate, and in how they co-accomplish safety.

Observational and participative safety research

Studying the ways in which particular treatments are delivered enables us to clarify and enhance their *in situ* enactment. For example, by monitoring the extent to which practitioners follow existing guidelines (Lingard *et al.*, 2005) and facilitating staff to systematise their practices (Campbell *et al.*, 1998), we may be able to simplify to some extent what practitioners do in the here and now. Simplification is an important aim, even when studies of how procedural guidelines and checklists are used in practice reveal that the complexity of *in situ* work frequently overwhelms practitioners' attempts to apply and stick to simple rules and procedures (Bosk *et al.*, 2009).

Another strand of research investigates how practitioners handle *in situ* demands and what resources they mobilise to cope with such demands. Homing in on complexity, this type of research is carried out using ethnographic approaches (Bergs *et al.*, 2005; Michaelson and Levi, 1997; Santora *et al.*, 1996). Typical of this alternative kind of research is close attention to *in situ* practice and the complexities it harbours (Mesman, 2009). Here, the analyst reveals the risks affecting practice, or the resources dynamically mobilised by practitioners for doing safety (Mesman, 2011).

Yet another strand of research promotes the involvement of practitioners in the study of *in situ* practice, and preferably their own practice. Involvement is advocated on the view that practitioners embody important knowledge and insight about their own practices, that such knowledge and insight form a critical basis for workplace learning, and that such learning is superior to information dissemination, which forms the basis of the other kinds of research. Orienting this participatory research are four assumptions.

1. Work is by definition complex because it is not linear and fully predictable.
2. Information about such work will forever remain partial and incomplete.
3. The practitioner will need to devise new knowledge, information, solutions and actions on the spot as part of a dynamic team and evolving task definition arrangement.
4. The group or team needs to have deliberative capability or 'distributed intelligence' for re-negotiating and reinventing their collective competences.

Involving practitioners in the research advocated here means focusing on locality and specificity. For many, to delve into the specifics of 'what goes on here' is to sacrifice generality and forfeit generalisation (Greenhalgh *et al.*, 2011). Generalisation is still regarded as the cognitive and scientific manoeuvre par excellence. This is on the assumption that when something holds true at time A in place X, it will hold true at time B in place Y, thanks to the power of generalisation. What we know about complex processes, however, is that what holds true in one place and time need not apply later and elsewhere. If it does apply later and elsewhere, it is unlikely to do so in its original form. For that reason, knowledge about complex phenomena is by definition uncertain (Prigogine, 1996).

Research is therefore obliged to extend its focus from 'generating knowledge about' to 'intervening in the *in situ* dynamics of knowing'. This reorientation heralds a new and different research paradigm. Our ambition now is not principally to generate generalities that are assumed to guide future action. This is 'producing knowledge about what works'. Rather, we seek to enmesh research in how practitioners act and learn amidst complexity. This is 'engendering new ways of doing, saying and knowing'. We favour the latter because acting amidst complexity is less about applying stable knowledge, than about coping with the dynamics of ongoing knowing, and learning about how to go on in uncertain situations.

Here we ask, how can we position ourselves in relation to others such that we maximise our chance of finding out what we need to know to be able to go on? This is less a matter of 'known knowledge', than about reading an evolving situation that demands constant updating about who does, says and knows what.

The question about how to position ourselves amidst uncertainty is a practical one. It correlates with a number of more general and perhaps more philosophical questions: What is it like to work under conditions of uncertainty? What does pervasive uncertainty mean for our professional identity? What status do we accord to that delicate and unpredictable process of 'coming to know' as and when practice unfolds? What does practice improvement mean when circumstances are increasingly emergent, complex and unpredictable?

Research that asks, 'how do clinicians position themselves?' inevitably also has to confront these more philosophical questions. The only way to answer any of these questions however is by considering how clinicians communicate.

As noted in the previous chapter, communication encompasses what we say to one another, but it involves other kinds of meaning-making too: gesture, facial expression, bodily comportment, and so forth, and also writing, and other technologically mediated forms of communication (diagrams, monitor displays,

X-rays, etc.). For practitioners, many of these aspects of communication are so embedded in their ways of working that they regard them as taken-as-given. This is in part because these aspects appear so subservient to the more important task of going through the surgery list, meeting the 4- or 6-hour emergency department access target, and so forth.

The communication dimensions of these superordinate activities are taken for granted also because of the lack of opportunity that practitioners have for paying attention to their own and each other's conduct. This renders moment-to-moment conduct the seemingly neutral, transparent medium through which we do more important things: diagnosis, treatment, assessment, and so on. And yet, moment-to-moment conduct and the communication that realises it are critical to the quality (and safety) of the technical-clinical processes of diagnosis, treatment, and assessment.

True, there is an increasing use of video feedback during clinicians' training years, particularly for technical skills but also increasingly for practising non-technical skills. But once at work, and some notable exceptions notwithstanding (Broekhuis and Veldkamp, 2007; Kaiser Permanente, 2010; Neuwirth *et al.*, 2012), clinicians receive little to no training in observing or paying attention to the lived dimensions of their own practices, let alone the lived dimensions of quality and safety.

Revealing the lived dimensions of safety engages people – researchers and clinicians alike. Without such engagement we have but limited understanding of how and why clinicians act as they do, and we have few clues about why or how to achieve change. Ethnography is critical to researching safety as practice, because it anchors the researcher(s) to the lived dimensions of *in situ* practice – the specificities of how clinicians enact knowing in practice. This needs to be complemented with a participative element, to prevent ethnography's close attention to what professionals do becoming a self-satisfied, objectifying and 'academic' exercise.

Participative research introduces a range of checks and balances to prevent ethnography from objectifying what clinicians do. It creates a blurring of roles between the researcher who observes and the practitioner who is observed. By allowing the practitioner a say in the relevance of the observational data gathered, the researcher may reflect on their *own* strategies and assumptions. By allowing the practitioner to view and question the observational data, they are enabled to evaluate such data in relation to how they understand their own work processes. It is at this participative intersection that researching safety connects with doing safety, and vice versa. Here, the gap that haunts the 'implementation of evidence into practice' is circumvented, knowledge and practice are short-circuited, and finding, insight and motivation for change coincide.

Finally, the approach to research just described embeds and manifests complexity thinking and complexity talking. It does so by acknowledging that the common practice of maintaining an objective distance and producing research knowledge *in abstracto* needs to be counterbalanced by a new and more dialogic research paradigm. This new paradigm allows – no, *capitalises* – on closeness, on meshing researcher and practitioner interests and practices.

Conclusion

This chapter has explained why and how the research advocated here engages with front-line clinicians. Why: in order to clarify the complexity and the logic of how they 'do safety'. How: involving clinicians in observing and reflecting on observational data. In this, engagement is critical and central. Researcher proximity to how clinicians work reveals both the dynamics and the distributed or networked nature of clinicians' decision-making, their communication and their activity generally. Clinician proximity to the research enables them to capitalise on the reflexive potential of observational data.

With this, we turn the Enlightenment 'ideal' of objectivity on its head. This is because complexity renders anything that may seem 'objective' short-lived. Where traditional twentieth-century approaches to health services research and practice improvement privileged objective knowledge at the expense of hunches and intuitions, twenty-first century approaches acknowledge that complexity demands fast feedback communication and creativity. Here, fast and innovative feedback more so than long-established disciplinary convention determines what is worth doing, saying and knowing.

Part of this 'turn to feedback' is a temporal and spatial shrinking. Our focus is increasingly on the details of *in situ* practice. This is because the formal resources, expert knowledges and existing procedures are realised *in situ*, from moment to moment. To really understand safety, we believe, we need to understand how practitioners act in the here and now. Equally important however is that practitioners themselves understand and observe how they themselves act in the here and now. Our concern with the here and now is thus not to objectify it by fixing how we experience and name it. Instead, we want to give it new value and momentum, both among those studying work and those doing the work.

Put differently, we are not concerned in this book to objectify safety, and turn it into some kind of formal, generalised knowledge about what works. We know that, in practice, safety is as likely to be a dynamic, creative, non-linear and opportunistic activity, as an 'objective', predictable one.

In this chapter we introduced a number of technical terms. One such term was 'adaptive practice': the way in which practice shapes itself and is shaped to emerging circumstances. Adaptive practice requires social or 'distributed intelligence'. Distributed intelligence points to the speed of feedback among practitioners. The more frequent and quicker the feedback, the more opportunities for adaptation, and the more intelligent, or healthy, or effective, the practice. Equally, the more frequent and quicker the feedback, the better the team will be at handling the future, or what we termed 'futurising the present'. All these phenomena are complex, and they are communication-based.

When we consider the clinical work close up, we see clinicians constantly searching for meanings, opportunities and possibilities. They do so surrounded by incomplete or uncertain information and inconsistent practices and models. Since the production of safety involves making safety trade-offs among all kinds of information, knowledge, interests, concerns, constraints and opportunities, our enquiry into safety cannot risk distancing itself from how these manifest as on-the-ground dynamics. In that regard, the notion 'participation' takes on a double significance. Safety research does not just require the enquirer to participate (as researcher) in practice, but also requires the practitioner to participate (as practitioner) in the enquiry.

4

Exnovation

Innovation from within

Introduction
················

Innovating handovers and ward rounds

SBAR stands for 'situation-background-assessment-recommendations'. SBAR is a handover protocol that was recently introduced into health care from defence. It makes explicit the kinds of information that people need to hand over from shift to shift, or from team to team (Haig *et al.*, 2006). Haig *et al.*'s (2006) publication rode the cusp of a wave of interest in clinical handover. Around the industrialised world, findings started to be published stating that inadequate handover communication plays a major role in incidents. In response, governments and agencies began to make funding available for clinicians and researchers to study clinical handover processes. Policies were issued requiring services to proceduralise clinical handover (Australian Commission on Safety and Quality in Health Care, 2009; London Ambulance Service, 2008; New South Wales Health, 2009). Literature reviews were published collating the evidence on clinical handover systematisation (Cohen and Hilligoss, 2010; Jorm *et al.*, 2009).

In their original and comprehensive overview, Cohen and Hilligoss (2009) list 19 handover acronyms. For their part, Riesenberg *et al.* (2009) list 24 acronyms. In Australia, SBAR was expanded into ISOBAR to accommodate the need for an Introduction and mention of Observations. This acronym was subsequently expanded into 'HAND ME AN ISOBAR' to accommodate preparation for the handover. HAND stands for 'Hey it's handover time; Allocate staff for continuity of patient care; Nominate participants, time and venue; Document by using handover sheet'. ME stands for 'Make sure all participants have arrived; Ensure leadership is provided during handover'. AN stands for 'Alert to special patient needs; Notice patient and staff movements and numbers'. ISOBAR stands for Introduction, Situation, Observations, Background, Assessment and Recommendation.

The 'HAND ME AN ISOBAR' phrase could well be expanded further. One suggestion is 'HAND ME AN ISOBAR, QUICKLY', where 'QUICKLY' acts as a reminder to 'Question the assessment and recommendations; Utilise the occasion to lecture juniors on the patient management plan; Interrogate them on their understanding of the case; Check their paperwork; Key main patient management changes into EMR; Last chance for comments and questions; and Yes, we've now finished!'

The 'QUICKLY' suggestion is not intended to make fun of acronyms. On the contrary, acronyms are handy ways for practitioners to seal an agreement and perpetuate a shared understanding. But the question that nevertheless arises here is, will teams adopt these acronyms 'as is', or do they generally see a need to adjust them, perhaps even reinvent them to suit their own unique circumstances?

In our experience, once practitioners see the need for systematisation of what they do, they will do so in a way that suits them and their local circumstances. Therefore, they will tend to adapt existing acronyms (checklists, procedures or guidelines), or even develop their own (Iedema *et al.*, 2009d). Their solutions may be unique, but they also tend to harbour at least some similarity to 'off-the-shelf' solutions. Their uniqueness is important to give practitioners the sense that they have had a hand in shaping their own ways of working. Their similarity to general policy advice should reassure managers that bottom-up systematisation need not necessarily lead to unacceptable forms of practice variation.

What is critical in all this, ultimately, is not the solution itself, whether it be an off-the-shelf one or a newly designed one, but, rather, that practitioners have the ability to articulate and agree together how their work currently unfolds, and how it (or a particular aspect of their work) is to unfold (Iedema *et al.*, 2012b). This activity of articulating how their work should unfold is useful on several fronts: it will enable senior staff members to test their degree of shared understanding, it teaches juniors about how senior clinicians think, it enables everyone to revisit solutions if/when they are out of date, and it enables practitioners to address a host of other dimensions of their work that rely on carefully negotiated and communicated agreements for their continuity and safety.

The importance of such planning activity is that it enables practitioners to reflect on 'how do we do our work?' and 'what do we take as given?' It helps them identify and fix problems in a local, negotiated and dynamic way. It enables them to think systemically and practically at the same time, making their own moment-to-moment behaviours relevant to the system's or a procedure's operation. This is ultimately what 'flexible systematisation' of shared tasks and responsibilities is about and how it is achieved (Timmermans and Berg, 2003).[11] Practitioners don't just practise blindly; instead, they negotiate their ways of working through shared online and offline deliberation. Such deliberation may contribute to systematising practice in ways that are flexible, precisely because practitioners now have the capacity (the 'meta-discourse') for routinely revisiting, updating and extending existing work process solutions.

This chapter explains the basic premise of bottom-up systematisation. We refer to bottom-up systematisation as *exnovation*, or 'innovation from within'. Such innovation arises from *within* established practice, and from within practitioners', patients' and researchers' collective sense-making of that practice. As such, and without denying the usefulness of these things, what we propose here does not turn on external analysis conducted by researchers elsewhere, or patients' experiences whose implications will be worked out in due course, or practitioners' taking action in response to formal data representing their own practice. Rather, exnovation turns on a process of shared deliberation that springboards off experiential data: footage and stories about *in situ* care (Quaid *et al.*, 2010).

Experiential data enable practitioners and other stakeholders to reflect on how the care unfolds from moment to moment. Such data connect people to what they or those close to them do and say, and this forges a link between them (even if what they see leads them to critique others), and connects them to who they are, what they say, and what they witness in what they hear and see in the data. Here, what matters is not distance, analysis, impartiality and objectivity, but connection, interpretation, recognition and immediacy. In what follows, we will explain the theoretical and pedagogic basis of this paradigm of investigation and intervention.

To be sure, the process of involving people in reflecting on their own ways of working using video data is by no means unique (Hargie and Morrow, 1986; Jeffers and Guthrie, 1988). Indeed, video is used in many forms of clinical train-

---

11 Timmermans and Berg coined the term 'flexible standardisation'. We replace the term 'stand-ardisation' with 'systematisation' because central here are not measurement and evaluation, but regularisation and proceduralisation.

ing nowadays, particularly those using simulation.[12] As noted in the previous chapter, numerous opportunities now exist for novices and junior professionals to engage in video and narrative-based reflection. However, involving post-experience (senior) professionals in reflexive service and practice redesign is less common. Opportunities do exist in the form of clinical outcomes reviews, throughput target audits, and the like (Carroll and Edmondson, 2002). These activities serve to 'interrupt' routine practice by enabling practitioners to think about what they and their colleagues do at a more general level. Exnovation has much in common with these kinds of activities. It involves practitioners in taking time out from their routine work processes. It involves them in considering representations of work processes. It is contingent on senior leadership support. Also, it encourages practitioners to draw conclusions from what they see, and use these to intervene in their everyday ways of working. However, there are also some critical differences.

These commonalities with existing processes of clinical redesign notwithstanding, exnovation adopts a very different approach to learning and pedagogy. Its pedagogy privileges what practitioners *do* in their day-to-day work. Their day-to-day work is not framed in statistics, but it is replayed as much as possible as it happens or as it is experienced. In doing so, we resist drawing conclusions on the basis of predetermined systems of measurement and calculation. Instead, we connect with people's sense of what happens or happened.

As we clarify shortly, most learning theories, including that of 'transformative learning' (Mezirow, 1997), target cognitive structures such as 'mental models' or 'cognitive frames of reference'. These theories are most concerned with *individuals'* attitudes and beliefs. But there are other learning theories that do not place the single individual at the centre of what happens (Gergen, 2009). These theories pay attention to what people *do* together, rather than what individuals think, believe and know. This shift in focus is in recognition of, on the one hand, the fact that collective action has a quality that cannot be fully explained with reference to, or as the sum of, individuals' intentions, knowledge, attitudes and beliefs. On the other hand, human practice encompasses a host of non-human phenomena (tools, technologies, resources) that shape people's actions, over and above their personal knowledge and individual intentions.

---

12 Hitchock *et al.* (2003) note:

> Interventions using video self-modeling began to appear in the literature in the early 1970s. Creer and Mildich (1970) introduced the term self-modeling when they reported using a videotape of a boy who was hospitalized with asthma role-playing effective social skills. The results showed that role-playing had no effect on behavior but viewing the videotape did.

For these reasons, exnovation concerns itself first and foremost with *existing kinds of activity*, or with what practitioners do together as they engage in practice. In targeting everyday activity and relationships, exnovation harbours commonalities with appreciative enquiry and participatory research, but it also offers crucial differences. What uniquely defines exnovation is its reliance on group-based reflexivity using experiential resources, such as video footage of *in situ* practice. In that regard, exnovation harnesses collectivist learning theory to interventionist research practice.

In what follows, we elaborate these points. We start with a definition of exnovation and an overview of its pedagogical underpinnings (*see* next section, 'Defining exnovation'). Then, in the section 'Exploring "what is"' (p. 80), we describe the collaborative practices that come into play when social science researchers work with front-line clinicians and patients to effect exnovation. Here, we refer to the investment that everyone needs to make in exnovation to ensure it touches base with the richness and complexity of existing practices, rather than gauge practice against regulatory standards, or scrutinise it only where and when it lapses into failure. We conclude the chapter with the section 'Exnovation as (social) science' (p. 88), which discusses the *politics* of exnovation. Here we consider how exnovation's capacity for short-circuiting insight and instigating change can perturb and unsettle existing relationships, practices and understandings.

Defining exnovation

Building on De Wilde (2000), we began this book with defining exnovation as follows. Exnovation foregrounds the actual and potential richness hidden in everyday activity and front-line staff relationships. Exnovation guides us to probing how clinicians communicate and act as a collectivity and how they make their work safe as a collectivity (Gherardi and Nicolini, 2002; Klein, 1999; Weick and Roberts, 1993). Exnovation seeks to describe the 'distributed' dimensions of practice – the ways in which practitioners' collective competence (Boreham *et al.*, 2000) enables them to co-create a *weave of safe care*. Exnovation throws light on the warp and weft of that weave, showing what it is that practitioners do to accomplish continuous and coherent patient treatment. Rendering this warp and weft explicit opens up the opportunity for transforming the group's tacitly held collective competence into a more articulate kind of distributed intelligence.

Highlighting the structure of that weave may of course reveal cracks. Cracks may happen when clinicians' activities are discontinuous, fragmented or conflicting (Manidis and Scheeres, 2012). However, no practice is likely to be without cracks, and paying close attention to what people do (not just what they say they do) will reveal strengths as well as opportunities for change. In suggesting that we should focus on what people *do* in the here and now, we signal that the approach advocated here is not a conventional one. To appreciate this, let us clarify our stance on 'what is' or our *ontology*; our view of 'how we know' or our *epistemology*, and our position on 'how we are to relate to others' or our *axiology*.

The attempt to understand what people do and make claims about what they do means establishing 'what is'. This is an ontology of practice. To ask about ontology is to seek answers to the question, what is going on? Instead of concerning itself with individuals' attitudes, values, and beliefs, a practice ontology wants to confront the complexities of *in situ* activity. This includes inspecting what people do, what resources they use, the cracks in what they do and the outcomes produced by what they do (Schatzki, 2005).

The truth status attributed to our claims, knowledge and representations is defining of our epistemology. Epistemology seeks answers to the questions, what is the basis of what we know, how do we come to know and how firm is our knowledge? The following is a typical *epistemological* claim: many people regard statistical representations as offering an unproblematic view of 'the real', and they give these representations a high truth status. Another epistemological claim is to say, all representations are constrained, albeit in different ways. None of them can fully capture everything there is to know about the real (Eco, 1984). While video footage, narratives and statistics are similarly constrained, video and narratives highlight conflicts, contradictions and dynamics – things that numerical data tend to erase from view. For that reason, video and narratives make possible a different way of knowing 'the real'. They derive from a different epistemological standpoint.

Finally, the ethical norms and values we feel we need to adhere to as humans form the basis of our axiology. Axiology pertains to how we feel we should relate to others. Video and narrative highlight how people feel and how they act, aside from what they say. This offers a possibility for rapprochement, enabling people to reassess what goes on with regard to lived experience, not just formal calculation. An axiological claim is to say, video enables people to go beyond conventional ways of relating, and it thereby opens things up, taking people beyond traditional ways of framing what is done and how. Another axiological claim is to say, it is ethical to enable people to reconsider how they relate, because doing so may give people the opportunity to reframe and revalue what is done. It may mean their concerns can be made to play a role in how matters are discussed, and in what judgements and measurements are applied.

In suggesting that practitioners need a say in defining 'what is', we acknowledge that ontology is contingent on different people's views and experiences – it is not a natural given, an 'out there' that can be established once and for all. In suggesting that knowledge arises from what different people can tell each other, and that it can change depending on who is present and how they share it with each other, we distance ourselves from a more traditional epistemology that views knowledge as independent from the individuals who articulate it. Traditional epistemology regards knowledge as truthfully reflecting the real out there, thereby making it incontrovertible.

In suggesting we need to collaborate with those who are the 'subjects' in our study, we advocate an axiology, an *ethics*, of relationships and collaboration. We leave aside research that excludes subjects from its design, data identification and analysis. We do so in the knowledge that 'scientific objectivity' can never be absolute and is inevitably always relative to specific people's interests and concerns. We do so also knowing that subjects' involvement enriches research outcomes. Finally, in according subjects a role in developing knowing, and linking this to their ability to change practice, we adopt the position that learning is not a matter of transforming individuals' mental models, but of engaging people in a practice of deliberation, a shared reflexivity, and in practical experimentation (Dewey, 1922).

The main influences of this book

This book's main influences derive from educational philosophy, science and technology studies, recent approaches to organisational learning, contemporary research methodology, and critical approaches to health care practice improvement.

Thus, the idea that the potential for innovation lies within existing practices (or 'habits') was strongly articulated in John Dewey's educational philosophy (Dewey, 1922, 1944). This principle has been central to Yrjö Engeström's work on organisational learning (Engeström, 2008) as well as Silvia Gherardi's (Gherardi, 2007) and Davide Nicolini's work (Nicolini, 2011). Paul Bate's (2000) account of health organisational change introduced the 'innovation-from-within' concept to health care practice improvement.

Closely related to these endeavours is that of *transformative research and evaluation* (Mertens, 2009). Working with marginalised communities, Donna Mertens advocates close collaboration between researchers and the 'subjects' of research. Related endeavours are Cooperrider and Whitney's 'appreciative enquiry' (Cooperrider and Whitney, 1999), and Reason and Bradbury's (2008) 'participative

---

enquiry', both of which give prominence to exploring the norms and reasoning underpinning existing practices instead of positioning critique as the principal aim and outcome of research.

These approaches intersect with Rouch's (2003) and MacDougall's (2006) 'participatory video-making'. Participatory video-making has since been extended from a collaborative production of documentary into a collaborative approach to producing visual feedback resources for kick-starting social or community deliberation about critical issues and unspeakable problems (Thomas, 2011).

The deliberative dimension of the present work also makes quite a bit of use of first-person narration, which anchors it to Trish Greenhalgh and colleagues' 'narrative-based improvement' (Greenhalgh *et al.*, 2005; Martin, 2011).

A critical influence to mention is science and technology studies. Marc Berg's work on the complexities of systematising medical work and the enablements and constraints inscribed into guidelines and protocols has been a defining influence on the present book (Berg, 1997, 1998; Berg and Mol, 1998). Timmermans and Berg's (2003) 'flexible standardisation' inspired our notion of 'flexible systematisation'. 'Flexible systematisation' emphasises we are not concerned in the first instance with making practitioners meet standards and benchmarks, but with engendering practitioner awareness of existing and potential systems of practice.

Last, but by no means least, Bruno Latour's work underpins our interest in how actors perform sociality into being (Latour, 2005). Latour informs our focus on 'matters of concern' rather than 'matters of fact' (Latour, 2004). John Law's and Annemarie Mol's exposition of the complexities of practice also provided much of the present book's critical philosophical groundwork (Law and Mol, 2002).

The foregoing suggests that exnovation is not in the first instance about change. It is in the first instance about observing and appreciating the way things *are*. This means confronting clinical work in all its complexity. In doing so, exnovation is not about creating a 'truer' picture of our complex world than we currently have, although it can make clinicians aware of matters they cannot see despite being deeply involved in the practice in question (Iedema *et al.*, 2007). Rather, exnovation is about engendering articulations, or expressions that frame for those involved aspects of their work that heretofore were allowed to remain invisible and therefore intangible.

In effect, exnovation is not concerned in the first instance with things that go wrong. This differentiates it from other approaches prevalent in health care research. Most start out from a 'deficit perspective'. That is, most health care research is intent on classifying and analysing problems and incidents as the route par excellence towards improvement (Mesman, 2011). The point of departure for exnovation, in contrast, is that what clinicians, patients and families do together is mostly adequate.

While rarely 'excellent', everyday practice is by and large effective in what gets accomplished, in the solutions it produces, in how often errors are averted, and in the resilience shown by people in the face of problems (Mesman, 2008; Wears *et al.*, 2008). Everyday clinical practice is underappreciated in so far as people's 'indigenous' (i.e. their own) insights and inventiveness are concerned. We still know little about how to capitalise on these capacities and energies. This may be thanks to our anxiousness to be seen to have 'the' answers: 'what works' guidelines and 'how to' checklists. Then, when things go wrong, we are preoccupied with incidents and investigations, at the expense of paying attention to the moment-to-moment unfolding of care, and all the resources mobilised by those doing the care.

For its part, exnovation does not 'objectify' what people believe and do. Popular ways of capturing employees' 'safety attitudes' include survey questionnaires, incident reports and analyses of incident investigations (Runciman *et al.*, 2007). These methods impose predetermined classifications, reinforcing classifiers' own views of the world. In contrast, exnovation seeks to produce insight into the *in situ* accomplishment of safety. It does so by asking practitioners to 'put themselves at risk' by letting themselves be videoed or videoing themselves, by observing themselves and each other at work (Iedema *et al.*, 2006), or by watching patients talking about their experiences of their care (Bate and Robert, 2007).

Common objections to video-reflexivity as practice improvement approach: rebutted

Objections have been raised about using video footage for practice improvement. First, there is the *arbitrariness* objection. Because a camera or any number of cameras can only be in one or some places at a time, video footage shows only what a very small number of practitioners happen to be doing at a particular time and in a particular place. It is impossible to film all relevant aspects of practice all of the time. For these reasons, it is claimed, video is incapable of revealing anything but strictly local and coincidental activities. No amount of video footage can be representative of all the relevant aspects of practice. Therefore, video does not provide a suitable means for achieving practice improvement.

Those who mount this objection fall prey to a naïve view of reality. That is, they regard 'reality' as a totality of 'goings-on' and understand effective action on that 'reality' to be conditional on our understanding of this totality. This objection founders on the following two considerations. One, were 'reality' to be conceived as a single, overarching totality of 'goings-on', apprehending it would necessitate 'a point of view from nowhere'. The 'point of view from nowhere' is logically impossible and the 'single reality' idea, therefore, is incoherent (Nagel, 1989). Two, there are numerous cultural manifestations of ongoing change in how humankind views and enacts 'the real'. This too indicates that the expectation of a comprehensive and complete perspective on 'the real' is not possible. It follows that humans command but a partial and incomplete view of/on 'the real'. All their attempts to know 'the real' – no matter how scientific – remain partial and incomplete. Albeit for different reasons, this partiality and this incompleteness are true both of large-sample-size studies and of single-case studies. The fact that video presents a partial and incomplete view of the real therefore does not constitute sufficient reason to reject it.

A second and frequent objection is that the use of the camera entrains the 'Hawthorne effect'. Here, it is claimed practitioners are so affected by the presence of the camera and by the knowledge they are being videoed that they end up significantly modifying (read: enhancing) how they do their work. However, in practice, and as those who have used video in workplaces can attest, people do not know very well how to act differently from what they do normally. If they do know how to enhance what they do, they are never able to maintain this for very long. They may take more care for a while to be seen to be doing the right or the appropriate thing, but in most cases people soon lapse back into their taken-as-given behaviours. This is because people are incapable of instant dis- and re-habituation (Dewey, 1922).

It is possible of course that the camera instils a consciousness in those videoed that differs from how they might otherwise apprehend themselves in practice. We certainly believe that altered awareness comes into play *after* participants have observed themselves at work (Iedema *et al.*, 2009e). It should be observed that the principal aim of the video-reflexive approach advocated here is altered awareness through altered relationships. This amounts to saying that the Hawthorne effect should not be regarded as a problem, but as the principal enabling factor underpinning and consolidating the effect of video-reflexivity.

Third, people object that you might film an incident, and that the incident footage can be subpoenaed by lawyers. This indeed is possible. The curious assumption that underpins this objection is that it is per definition 'bad' to have footage of an incident. Let us first state however that in our 10 years of filming acute care practice, we filmed one such incident (but it never was subpoenaed): three junior emergency department doctors stood deliberating about what to do while a woman had full-body muscle contractions and clearly needed attention to prevent her from dying. The footage might have been used to prove liability on the part of the junior doctors for not initiating some kind of treatment, or for not calling in a medical emergency team. The footage could equally well have been used to exonerate them. The chaos around them was such that even the most seasoned doctor or nurse would have been challenged in their attempt to save the woman. A number of patients needed urgent attention, and the department clearly lacked the requisite number of senior clinicians.

Consider, too, that incidents do not come out of the blue: they build up from the actions of different individuals over time and across sites. Such incidents are near impossible to film. Further, the objection that you might film an incident and therefore should not use video also falters on the consideration that footage of *in situ* work can *alleviate* rather than support allegations of responsibility and liability. This is because video captures the rich context within which individuals provide care: the host of factors that influence or affect what people do and say. Knowing that most clinicians do not intend to harm their patients, we believe that video footage contains portrayals of contextual factors that might actually support clinicians' claim they were trying their best, instead of containing additional evidence for their liability.

Finally, if something goes wrong in health care, we would expect those involved to *want* to know as much as possible about how it happened. It may be advantageous to have footage of what happened. To assume that video footage is likely to confirm practitioners' liability is to assume that such people *are* likely to be liable. To reject the use of video on this basis, besides suggesting that one would be prepared to bury liable practice, is to deny that professionals have an obligation towards patients to learn from incidents and prevent them from happening again. Therefore, 'you might video-film an incident' is not a credible objection. Defining of professionalism, surely, is confidence in one's standards and in one's willingness and ability to learn from incidents. In our experience, it is indeed those clinicians who are confident and curious who sign up to being videoed.

Video-based 'reflexive' processes make what is otherwise experienced as normal and mundane appear novel and strange (Garfinkel, 1972). What makes things strange is seeing (or hearing) the things we are familiar with 'from under a different aspect' (Wittgenstein, 1953). We hear people describing those things in terms that are personal to them but which may be strange to us. We watch ourselves doing things from an unusual angle, and on a small screen. 'Making the normal strange' (O'Toole and Shukman, 1977) unhinges us from our taken-as-given world, from our accepted self, and from the habits that buttress and insulate that world and that self.

Making these things strange may unsettle people. However, as Peter Sloterdijk insists, our contemporary world is now so complex that it demands from us the capability to apprehend ourselves and our actions from under a different aspect (Sloterdijk, 2009). This is because doing so produces new kinds of dialogue, new questions, and new possibilities for being, insight and action – all necessary for acting amidst complexity. In this way, making the normal strange is critical to our participation in an increasingly complex world (Sloterdijk, 2009).

Acting amidst complexity, for Sloterdijk, is contingent on our capacity to apprehend 'what is' in new ways. He refers to this capacity to apprehend 'what is' as our 'passivity competence'. Passivity competence is the competence to be open to what is happening around us and to what others are doing, enabling us to respond to it rapidly.

> Indeed, passivity competent conduct belongs to the play/game intelligence that defines all people living in the contemporary networked world, where we cannot make a move without also being moved. (Sloterdijk, 2009: 594)[13]

Exnovation is about being moved by what might otherwise appear to be mundane and taken as given. For that reason, exnovation is about *affect*. This is not in the first instance about knowing more, but about knowing differently by making things visible in different ways. This may be achieved through videoing practice and through deliberation about the resulting footage with others. This is why we regard the process and outcome of exnovation as turning on a shared and sharable intelligence.

This is a critical point. Exnovation is not a technique that enables experts elsewhere to accumulate formal knowledge upon which to base new directives. Exnovation also does not subscribe to social science's favourite activities: analysing and deconstructing practices and discourses, laying bare their structure and privileges, and mounting criticisms and critiques 'from a distance'. This is what Latour refers to as 'pulling the rug from underneath people' (Latour, 2004). Instead, exnovation works through *affect*, through relationships that enable

---

13 This is our translation from the original German, which reads: 'In Wahrheit gehört das passivitätskompetente Verhalten zur Spielintelligenz von Menschen in einer entfalteten Netzwelt, in der man keinen eigenen Zug machen kann, wenn man nicht zugleich mit sich spielen läßt.'

participants to do and say new things about the familiar and taken-as-given, as well as about the challenging and unpredictable that permeates practice.

An example of this competence is found in the following description of a planning meeting where participants engage in 'collective creativity', or 'bricolage':

> In their most productive moments, participants in consensus building engage not only in playing out scenarios, but also in a kind of collective, speculative tinkering, or bricolage . . . That is, they play with heterogeneous concepts, strategies and actions with which various individuals in the group have experience, and try combining them until they create a new scenario that they collectively believe will work. This bricolage . . . is a type of reasoning and collective creativity fundamentally different from the more familiar types, argumentation and trade-offs . . . Bricolage . . . produces, rather than a solution to a known problem, a new way of framing the situation and of developing unanticipated combinations of actions that are qualitatively different from the options on the table at the outset. The result . . . is, most importantly, learning and change among the players, and growth in their sophistication about each other, about the issues, and about the futures they could seek. (Innes and Booher, 1999: 12)

Exnovation is about 'learning and change among the players, and growth in their sophistication about each other, about the issues, and about the futures they could seek' (Innes and Booher, 1999: 12). To make such learning and change possible, players need 'passivity competence'; that is, the ability to put stock conducts and answers on hold, to defer routine responses, to query existing practice and knowledge, and to legitimate new kinds of answers and solutions. This competence is the precondition for players to achieve a weave of shared attention, manifested as 'a new way of framing the situation and of developing unanticipated combinations of actions that are qualitatively different from the options on the table at the outset' (Innes and Booher, 1999: 12).

Exnovation, then, is about engendering communicative openness. A precondition for such openness is passivity competence, or the capacity to allow others and other things to intervene in your and others' practice, thinking and self. Passivity and openness are critical for engaging with the full complexity of what goes on, without prejudging it and lapsing into routines and moves that are out of sync. This underscores that exnovation is not in the first instance about identifying knowledge, rules or truths, but about partaking in a deliberative process, in a forum of engagement.

Likewise, deliberation is not principally about reproducing what has been done and what is known, but about exploring what has not yet been done and what is not known. It requires the competence to consider existing relationships, identities and practices 'from under a different aspect'. We contend that this competence – 'seeing oneself, others and practices from under a different aspect' – is, in the final analysis, defining of health care safety (Iedema, 2011).

Exploring 'what is'

For most health services researchers the main objective is to mechanise both their own research processes and the clinical processes they choose to study. They do so through imposing strict research protocols which serve the production of strict clinical protocols or 'forcing functions' (Norman, 1988). The argument in favour of this 'command and control', top-down approach to safety (research) is that even the smartest clinician and the best-functioning team will eventually be defeated by the context in which they work, whether this be a poorly functioning system, others' slips and errors, or their own lapses. They need to know how the best among us would have acted. Certainly, being able to fall back on general rules may help practitioners navigate through complex situations. However, it does not enable them to be more than just reactive.

There is also little doubt now that front-line staff play a crucial role in preventing errors through their 'error wisdom' (Reason, 2004) – a special kind of insight that emerges from 'personal heedfulness' (Weick and Roberts, 1993) and 'social mindfulness' (Weick, 2004). Working their way through complex situations further brings out practitioners' ability to invent on-the-spot solutions, also referred to as resilience (Hollnagel, 2006). These characteristics enable employees to respond to and anticipate problems. Much safety issues from these kinds of conducts, but of course people are not always aware of the extent to which their own habituations predispose them, their colleagues and their patients to unsafety. In our view, therefore, safety is contingent on three things: (1) forcing functions, (2) resilience and (3) exnovation.

Clearly, forcing functions (think of guidelines, checklists, managerial directives) provide appropriate and well-studied routes for practice and behaviour. Equally, they can turn inappropriate routes into non-options through the technology or procedure not allowing error-prone actions, or through sign-off and read-back providing compulsory checks. Forcing functions are crucial to optimising the chance that, in situations where there are inadequate skill levels or excessive risk, safe routines will be followed. Complementing such forcing functions, employees' insight may help intercept many incidents about to happen and reduce them to 'near misses'.

All the while, however, day-to-day practice unfolds in a space that Amalberti and colleagues refer to as *normal–illegal*: a mode of practice that aligns with what is possible, more than with what is formally required (Amalberti *et al.*, 2005). In fact, the normal–illegal space of activity is made up of workarounds, shortcuts, and other not formally sanctioned or managerially endorsed actions. Amalberti's work suggests that there remains considerable discretionary space where the clinician needs to work out what requires (special) attention, and what forcing functions should be obeyed or mobilised and how (in cases where this is not automatic or self-evident). To operate in this discretionary space the practitioner has to rely on *phronesis* – 'practical know-how' (Bourdieu, 1990; Flyvbjerg, 2001). This know-how – this *phronesis* – is the principal focus and target of exnovation.

Phronesis is a notion coined by Aristotle for whom practice represented a dynamic fusion of *techné* (technical 'knowing-that'), *epistemé* (social-moral knowing) and *phronesis* (practical 'knowing-how'). We should not overestimate the role of knowing, however. As we learned from John Dewey, much human knowing is embedded in *habits*. This means that our use of knowing should not be taken to mean: I consciously apply my knowledge to a situation and deduce the correct action before I execute that action. On the contrary, my action is most likely to be structured on the basis of existing practices: what goes on around me, and what others do and have done over time. Dewey believes that very few of our actions and practices are consciously reasoned and fully planned (Dewey, 1922). In fact, much practical reasoning and planning is post hoc, after the fact, as if to legitimate what we would have done in any case (Damasio, 1994, 2003). On this view, many actions and practices are habituations that have been handed down to us by previous generations and people around us. This has led anthropologists to make so much of 'culture', a term they use to describe the peculiar and often arbitrary nature of what people do.

For clinical professionals this means the following. Generally, clinicians are inducted into their work in a vocational manner, with their educational curricula offering limited overlap with the practical dimensions of their work (Benner, 1994; Bloom, 1989). The practical – phronetic – dimension of the clinical work remains invisible until the learner enters health care employment. This invisibility of what you need to know to do the work has led commentators to coin the expression 'hidden clinical curriculum' (Bernstein, 1975; Bleakley, 2006).

What remains hidden is the practical logic that directs practical action. What the curriculum makes explicit is only formal scientific knowledge (Evans, 2008).

Let us frame this problem in another way. The yardstick by which junior *and* senior clinicians' credentials are measured targets explicit knowledge of scientific, clinical and ethical facts. What clinicians do on a moment-to-moment basis is rarely subjected to learning, except perhaps when they are still in training, do targeted simulation, or when things go wrong.

This state of affairs is detrimental for three reasons. First, it deprives clinicians of the opportunity to discuss aspects of their work that are effective, extraordinary, troubling or traumatic. This deprives them of the opportunity to determine what their experiences mean for how they do their work (Iedema *et al.*, 2009a). This situation also denies clinicians the opportunity to collectively develop a discourse with which they can discuss, creatively redesign and thereby systematise their own ways of working (Timmermans and Berg, 2003).

Furthermore and most problematically, this situation denies clinicians the opportunity to build relationships that are intelligent, because based on mutual regard, interpersonal support and a shared responsibility (Hutchins and Klausen, 1998). In effect, novices find themselves in the difficult position of having to work out what clinical practice is about, and how their formal knowledge relates to it (Shem, 1978). Ultimately, and most problematically, this disconnect between formal learned knowledge and *in situ* practice is the *condition of possibility* for Amalberti's 'normal–illegal' actions. That is, for as long as clinical practitioners fail to confront the *in situ* unfolding of their own work practices, will they remain oblivious to what actions are normal–illegal. This means they are also unlikely to recognise the junctures where their actions drift into the zone of the *dangerous*–illegal – the zone of error, failure and catastrophe (Dekker, 2011).

Safety, seen from our perspective, depends on communication about *in situ* activity ('what you and I do') and practice ('what and how things are done around here'). Safety is not just something we do in the here and now by being resilient in the face of problems and obeying forcing functions (the generalised obligations that pre-structure clinical routes and routines). Indeed, these two strategies are not primary but *secondary* to another one: clinicians building their *distributed intelligence* through testing their understandings with one another, sounding each other out about specific tasks and activities, and evaluating existing practices. This involves professionals in assessing and enhancing their team's safety sensibilities, and creatively communicating new work processes and practices into being. Central to building distributed intelligence too is regularly checking whether normal–illegal activities are drifting into a danger zone.

Communicating in the key of distributed intelligence – how do we accomplish our tasks from moment to moment, and how do we collectively do things around here – is central to our ability to orchestrate and reinvent safety in the here and now.

For these reasons, distributed intelligence is the principal target and aim of exnovation. How does distributed intelligence relate to phronesis? Well, phronesis becomes evident from what practitioners do in response to, for example, patient Smith in Bed 5 showing signs of deterioration, or the junior doctor appearing to have trouble with an intubation. However, only articulating their phronesis collectively enables practitioners to make visible and potentially reinvent their 'logic of practice' (Bourdieu, 1990). Talking about 'our logic of practice' nurtures distributed intelligence.

Of course, simulation enables people to articulate how and why they do things. Involving senior clinicians in simulation can be a powerful resource for strengthening their phronesis. Simulation however often prefigures what goes on and what is talked about – a team rescuing a deteriorating patient, a handover, a family conference, or an incident disclosure. These are valuable exercises. *In situ* practice, however, mobilises more complex kinds of conduct, and less common forms of phronesis.

To illuminate these, we need to take the time to explore, visualise and articulate what goes on *in situ*, the ordinary, moment-to-moment unfolding of clinical work. This enables us to discuss the taken-for-granted, the assumptions and experiences that we bring to bear on the work, the knowledge we have of how things are done here and elsewhere in the service, the sense we have of how others experience and respond to what we do, the concerns we have about the effectiveness of what goes on, and so forth. These articulations can be post hoc debriefs about a difficult event or set of events. They can also be ad hoc, addressing intuitions, concerns and new ideas.

What now is the relation between the articulation of this practical know-how and exnovation? In effect, exnovation is the process that kick-starts such communication. Exnovation's purpose is to enable practitioners to confront and articulate 'what is' – the team's current activities, processes, practices, experiences, feelings, concerns. This kind of discussion is not constrained by what the senior doctor and registrar know, or what the manager says must happen. This discussion addresses what *actually* goes on: the normal–legal, the normal–illegal, as well as the dangerous illegal. It can do this because the footage renders these things talkable. Footage shows us as practitioners all equally enmeshed in something bigger than 'just' our personal intentions and reasonings: practice. By foregrounding *practice* and backgrounding the individual, footage makes it possible for all involved, senior as well as junior people, to talk about how things are done.

Such discussion can address insights and uncertainties, questions and ideas. In that sense, such discussion becomes a safe place where we can talk about lingering doubts and concerns. As such, it creates a safe zone where we can share in asking and learning. Duscussion therefore becomes a 'zone of proximal development' (Vygotsky, 1986), or a 'zone of peripheral participation' (Lave and Wenger, 1990). These creative discussion zones are central to engendering distributed intelligence.

In such a safe zone, senior people can speak freely about how things are done and why. Speaking freely refers to a register that includes everyone present, and excludes pretending that things are better or more different than they are. Such register is critical to enabling senior staff to reassess the relative safety of practices, including taken-as-given illegalities. Novices can safely question activities and practices because it is acknowledged that their skills and expertise may not be optimal, and that their actions and utterances may not yet fully comply with the hidden rules that govern who they are and what they do. Such a safe zone requires and engenders flexibility, openness and bricolage. This is the condition of possibility for exnovation: a collective process that creates ideas and plans that are 'qualitatively different from the options on the table at the outset' (Innes and Booher, 1999: 12).

The politics of exnovation

Confronting professionals with what goes on and discussing how we do things is not at all straightforward. This is because it bares espoused understandings of what is true and right, and contrasts these with what in fact goes on. What in fact goes on includes not just workarounds, shortcuts, and normal–illegal activities, but also more arbitrary differences in practice born from divergent interpretations of guidelines, evidence and best practice. For instance, the vignette presented in Chapter 2 showed neonatal intensive care unit (NICU) doctors coming to the realisation that they do not see eye to eye on the relationship between necrotising enterocolitis and breast milk consumption.

Such divergent stances may be left implicit out of respect for individuals' professional autonomy, even if this renders everyday practice complicated for other team members. Initiating and facilitating conversations such as the one portrayed in the NICU vignette is by no means easy. The political and interpersonal ramifications of initiating such discussions can be far-reaching and sometimes unpleasant (Iedema *et al.*, 2004). We have experienced situations where senior personnel challenged other professionals' legitimacy, in an attempt to take away their right to have a say in the reflexive meetings. Such challenges need to be addressed immediately, and with great care. They should not go unquestioned. In such scenarios, a skilful outsider-facilitator is needed to ask questions that will expose the (il)logic underpinning such challenges, but which do so in a non-threatening way. Sometimes, interprofessional meetings can be hard to manage, but they are critical for working out how practice 'makes sense' to those enacting it (Iedema and Carroll, 2011).

To stay one step ahead of such political dilemmas, those pursuing exnovation need to be sensitive to the various positions that individual practitioners may articulate and defend. As a first step, everyone needs a say in the orientation and direction of the research. Achieving this avoids problems being studied (or not) to suit some stakeholders and not others. However, the negotiation of what is studied and how can be very challenging. The nurse unit manager may want to use the footage to ensure guideline compliance on the part of her nurses. The senior doctor may not want to focus on handover communication but target junior doctors' level of clinical comprehension. Here, delicate discussions are necessary to ensure the project maintains common ground.

A number of research approaches have been advocated that seek to involve practitioners in what the problems are to be studied, how they are to be analysed, and what is to be done with them and about them. Among others, cooperative enquiry (Reason, 1999) and appreciative enquiry (Cooperrider and Whitney, 1999) are participatory research approaches that give practitioners a voice in the orientation and outcomes of research:

> Participatory research . . . most clearly distinguishes itself from other forms of action-related research by the fact that it issues from the felt needs of the community. What motivates the initiation of participatory research is the needs of the community for ameliorating the living conditions of the people. (Park, 1999: 143)

Participatory research differs in subtle ways from 'ethnography', whose purpose is to portray the cultural practices of a group or community (Agar, 1980). Such portrayal relies on evidence whose principal yardstick is frequency of occurrence or 'saturation'. Saturation shields description from the charge of 'anecdotalism' (Anspach and Mizrachi, 2006). In that sense, ethnography is concerned with producing representative and defensible descriptions of practice. Participatory research inevitably delves somewhat further into everyday complexity, if only because it grants practitioners more say. Here, specific people's interests and accounts serve not just to map the contours of local complexity, but also to guide how we make sense of that complexity and how deeply we probe it.

No doubt, the main differences between these three approaches (ethnography, participatory research and appreciative enquiry) and exnovation are now coming into view. Exnovation differs from ethnography in that it does not presume to be able to generate a valid description ('-graphy') without involving those who are the focus of interest ('ethno-'). Exnovation differs from participative research in so far as it requires those who are the object of research interest to assume a research stance themselves, on themselves. Put differently, exnovation expects practitioners not just to participate in research discussions but to take the lead in such discussions. Exnovation differs from appreciative enquiry in that its point of departure is the engagement of the professional team with their *in situ* ways of working. These ways of working may be effective and worthy of appreciation; they may also be defective or politicised, in which case questioning and critique are in order.

However, through exnovation, and potentially facilitated by a researcher-outsider, practitioners themselves mobilise relevant questions and critiques. Exnovation thus centres on inspiring in professionals a reflexive capacity. Such capacity comes about through their re-evaluating their own practices and reasonings. Discussions in this register make manifest a team's *weave of shared intelligence*, with the quality of that weave defining the team's capacity for safety.

Here, we are a long way from the safety survey where individuals' responses to a decontextualised question are taken to have relevance for how such individuals act *in situ*, on the assumption that their beliefs and attitudes motivate how they act (Greatbatch *et al.*, 2001). There are many problems with the survey approach, the most prominent of which is not even the tenuous relationship between someone's espoused views, their formal responses, and their *in situ* actions. More problematic is the individualisation of safety, as if safety issues from individuals' heads.

Exnovation takes a very different stance. Safety is produced by collectives of professionals, and it is inherent in their weave of collaborative practice. These collectives produce safety by collectively confronting their *in situ* activities and practices, and by communicating reflexively about them. Exnovation is thus not just about participation, or about shared agenda setting, or about one's practices receiving appreciation, but about *taking over the research role*. This 'taking over' refers to professionals accepting responsibility for attending to the things they do day-to-day, and collectively re-creating and revitalising their shared intelligence. It should also be clear now that research is not merely about 'coming to know', but, perhaps more importantly, about 'enabling to do'.

The principal entry point for exnovation, therefore, is the creation of 'forums of engagement'. Such forums are sites where not matters of fact but matters of concern are raised and addressed (Latour, 2004). The shift from 'fact' to 'concern' is crucial here: it marks people's focus on apprehending practice, self and relations from different and contrasting points of view. That is, the value judgements that anyone in specific conventionally attaches to practice, self and relations are suspended, such that they can be juxtaposed with different and contrasting judgements. This is the political challenge of exnovation. Everyone, and not just those in authority, gets to say how they see themselves and their practice. Doing this opens us up to the complexity of the real in an entirely new and more forceful way, enabling us to reframe and redesign what we do, who we are, and how we relate to people.

This shows that exnovation is in the first place a *social* process bringing together researchers, clinicians, patient-consumers, managers and policymakers as stakeholders advocating their various concerns. By taking each other's concerns seriously, these players can come to different understandings of their world, and articulate new visions for that world. Exnovation drives this process as the means to engaging people with the complexity of their own practices, and, through that, the creation of alternative ways of being, saying and doing. The politics of this are complex, but what gives exnovation a unique advantage is its use of video data.

Video data anchor those participating in exnovation to a rudimentary record of practice: footage of people at work. While the angle of the camera and the choice of footage to be shown back to professionals are most definitely sensitive political choices that the researchers will be struggling with throughout the project (Iedema *et al.*, 2009e), the status of video footage as formal record of practice should keep in check professionals' tendency to veer off into expounding preferential knowledge and espoused opinions. Here, video footage of 'what happened' (albeit filmed from a particular angle and distance) serves as a leveller. The footage is to some extent incontrovertible. At the same time, it reveals *in situ* activity to be a bundle of taken-as-given routines and habituations whose reality and credibility are confirmed by people performing these routines as a matter of course. In that way, video foregrounds the social dimensions inherent in what we do, implicating us all.

This last point connects exnovation to the principle of 'just culture' (Dekker,

2008). The process of exnovation requires and realises trust among team members. Instead of trust being threatened by footage showing individuals to be doing unexpected, imperfect or illegitimate things, the socialising effect of video footage is to draw attention to people's shared responsibility for what is happening. Here, 'just culture' becomes tangible because, instead of holding each other personally responsible for what is going on, practitioners are obliged to acknowledge they are all caught up in and responsible for the unfolding of *in situ* activity. Exnovation further materialises the practice of leadership, another notion whose lofty principles often evade translation into concrete activities; by supporting and participating in exnovation, clinicians with seniority and authority show the way towards practice improvement, life-long learning and cross-boundary communication.

Exnovation as (social) science

Finally, exnovation is scientific, but not scientific in a Cartesian-Newtonian sense. Cartesian-Newtonian approaches to science are now judged to be subject to naïve-rational thinking (Russell *et al.*, 2008). Naïve-rational thinking demands absolute answers: something is either wholly true or not true. Such answers become possible thanks to large tracts of reality being excised from scientific consideration. As we explained in Chapter 3, Cartesian-Newtonian ways of thinking and doing science were challenged from their inception, but these challenges only fully came to prominence in the late nineteenth and early twentieth centuries when the 'hard sciences', i.e. physics and chemistry, no longer had any choice but to turn their gaze on themselves. What scientists like Heisenberg and Bohr observed was that their technical apparatuses, perceptual focus and philosophical underpinnings affected and even predetermined their findings. 'Out there' was no longer simply 'the real', but came to be seen as a complex effect of reality's material affordances and scientists' measurement technologies. Complexity entered science when scientific research was realised to *prefigure* its own research findings and scientific conclusions (Prigogine and Stengers, 1984).

Despite these developments in science, health research is still very much in the thrall of pre-complexity, naïve-rationalist scientific thinking (Russell *et al.*, 2008). This thinking manifests in the claim that there are 'gaps in knowledge' that can and must be filled. This terminology suggests that knowledge will accumulate until we know everything. But what in fact happens is that new knowledge only creates new uncertainties and ever-receding vistas (Prigogine, 1996).

Applied to social and organisational phenomena, conventional scientific approaches and knowledge tend to be too rigid and abstract to allow direct application and easy adaptation. Not surprisingly, those interested in complexity have begun to experiment with generating knowledge in ways that differ substantially from those that define formal, sanctioned research.

For its part, much social science has commonly assumed a critical agenda. Critique is a dominant characteristic of (medical) sociological kinds of enquiry.[14] Much sociological critique has sought to attack power and dominance, such as medicine's paternalistic treatment of patients, or the health system's inability to accommodate individual patients' preferences. To be sure, some of these studies have been groundbreaking. Notably, Illich's book, *Limits of Medicine* (Illich, 1976) offers a radical reversal of the propaganda that has driven medical science and practice since the days of William Osler, author of *The Principles and Practice of Medicine* (Osler, 1892). For Osler, medical progress

> effected a revolution in our civilisation . . . a revolution which for the first time in the history of poor, suffering humanity brings us appreciably closer to that promised day when the former things should pass away, when there should be no more unnecessary death, when sorrow and crying should be no more, and there should not be anymore pain. (Osler, 1892, cited in Bliss, 2011: 53)

In stark contrast, Illich's book starts with the sentence 'The medical establishment has become a major threat to health'. This threat, he argued, resulted from 'iatrogenic incidents', or medicine-caused harm. Four decades later, patient safety and health care incidents are (alongside access and resources) the most significant concerns in the minds of policymakers, managers, clinicians and patients. Equally influential, Glaser and Strauss' work showed that, in the 1960s, patients were not routinely informed by their doctor about the likelihood of their dying (Glaser and Strauss, 1965). Some years later they were able to show that this state of affairs had changed and that communicating about death and dying was becoming more common (Glaser and Strauss, 1968).

These notable examples of sociological-critical analysis notwithstanding, if critique becomes a driving research principle it also pre-assigns assumptions about the value of a practice and about the intentions of its practitioners. In satisfying its own critical agenda, such a stance may gloss over the complexities

---

14 Some of these studies practise critique by cynically appropriating a 'moral high ground' (Sloterdijk, 1984) and as such resemble the naïve-rational science that also claims to be able to occupy a 'point of view from nowhere' (Nagel, 1989) in matters of truth instead.

and uncertainties that permeate professional practice, such as contradictory reasoning, sub-conscious motivations, political tensions and competing responsibilities – the whole gamut of wicked problems and tragic circumstances that populate care. By downplaying the ways that wicked problems and tragic circumstances complicate care practices, and by misrecognising practitioners' dilemma in settling for taken-as-given habituations as best-possible responses, critique risks attributing an unrealistic degree of intentionality and control to health care professionals and policymakers – a degree of control which they possibly would like to have, but which in practice they will never have.

To repeat, this is not to say that critique has no place in research. What we do believe is that critique should neither be the single origin of nor the principal motivation for research. The principal motivation for the research promoted here is interested discovery, keeping judgements in abeyance until they emerge from a process of negotiation over what practice is, does, and means with all those who have a stake in the articulation of such judgements: researchers, professionals, managers, policymakers and patients. We advocate this because health care is too complex to abide quick judgements. Take the junior doctor who administered an overdose of insulin during the night, putting a patient's kidneys and potentially her life at risk. This trainee may well have acted as he or she did because of the illegibility of a senior doctor's medical record notation, their own fatigue due to long working hours, a lack of supervisory support, his or her fear of interrupting the senior consultant's night rest, a feeling of resignation on the part of the night nurse who cannot persuade the doctor to act otherwise, and responsibility avoidance from another clinician who wants to protect their specialty boundaries. In this scenario, as in most health care incidents, error, best practice, autonomy, politics, responsibility, accountability and disclosure all intertwine in complex ways.

Since scenarios such as this one are common, we need to militate against simple judgements, reductive conclusions and rapid criticisms (Dekker, 2008). For these reasons, the research advocated here promotes an approach that foregrounds local complexity. We believe that safety is achieved in the first and last instance by clinicians who do the work. The systems and resources that support them will never be optimal for all situations. Therefore, we take the complexity of *in situ* practice as our point of departure, and we harness the positive, affective energy that staff bring to their work to drive our research.

In the chapters that follow, we set out practical examples of how researchers and clinicians have put exnovation to use. We first turn to the example of how Katherine Carroll and Gordon Caldwell intervened in their respective departments' ward rounds. We then turn to the work of Jessica Mesman, Twan Mulder and Corine Kooyman in NICU in Maastricht University Medical Center to see how the use of video impacted on practice there. Next, we look at how Elizabeth van Rensen, Bas de Vries and Cor Kalkman motivated six hospitals to conduct video-ethnographic work focusing on post-operative handovers. Then, and finally, we hear about Chris Ball's and Rick Iedema's intervention enabling ambulance officers and emergency staff to settle on a handover protocol that ensures information that both parties find important is handed over. In our concluding chapter, we bring the various strands of our book together, summarising the special, unique and practical advantages of exnovation as a practice improvement method.

Section 2

5

Improving medical handover using video methodology

Two projects, two perspectives

Co-authored with Gordon Caldwell

Introduction

This chapter presents two practice-improvement projects that have used the video-reflexive methodology to achieve exnovation. Each project involved the videoing of doctors' ward round communications. In both projects, the doctors reviewed the footage to learn, evaluate and subsequently make changes for the betterment of communication. In both cases this process led to new insights and new practices in support of a more effective ward round. This chapter examines this process in detail. The focus is on ward round communication in two separate acute care units as case studies. The case studies demonstrate how clinicians and researchers can collaborate to exnovate the hidden or previously unrealised potential inherent in day-to-day clinical work.

In demonstrating how video-reflexivity works in practice, this chapter's case studies are presented by two very different professionals, both of whom took on the role of facilitator. The project reported on first was facilitated and videoed by a medical sociologist with a physiotherapy background, Katherine Carroll, working with a team of intensive care doctors. Being based at a university, Katherine occupied an 'outsider' role in relation to the intensive care medical team. Given her experience of hospital work, however, Katherine could also be considered an 'insider'. In that sense, she had the effect of a 'clinalyst' – a person whose function is to act as boundary-spanner (Iedema and Carroll, 2011). A clinalyst exposes insider knowledge to outsider questions, renders outsider insights part of insider knowledge, and encourages insiders asking questions of themselves and their colleagues.

The second project reported involved Gordon Caldwell videoing and reviewing a 'post-take ward round' in his acute medical unit. Gordon can be considered to be an 'insider' to the workings of both his team and the hospital, acting as an 'outsider' by introducing video as reflexive medium into his team's practice. In that sense, Gordon too functioned as a clinalyst, albeit approaching the task of boundary-spanning as it were from within, rather than from without, as Katherine did.

Taken together, these two case studies exemplify two important modalities of video-based exnovation. The first modality is that of the researcher 'outsider' working 'alongside' and in collaboration with front-line professionals organising and delivering care. The second modality is that of the 'insider' interested in practice improvement, focusing the camera on their own and on colleagues' practices. The chapter addresses the advantages and disadvantages of both stances in its concluding section. Overall, the chapter shows that through engaging visual methodologies, clinicians, researchers and managers come to sit alongside one another in the task of unravelling, challenging, celebrating, discussing and intervening in their practices.

A medical sociologist works alongside intensive care doctors to improve ward round communication

The first case study reported in this chapter takes place in an intensive care unit (ICU). The project focused on how intensive care clinicians create order in their work practices within their highly unpredictable organisational environment (Carroll, 2009; Carroll *et al.*, 2008). This involved observing and recording ICU clinicians' everyday work, interviewing clinicians formally about their work practices, and videoing a variety of routine work across nursing, medicine and allied health.

One focus was medical communication, particularly formalised communication such as the ward round. The ICU had two back-to-back sessions of formal medical communication every morning. The first occurred at 8 a.m., a ward round where the night staff handed over information to the oncoming day staff (*see*

Figure 5.1). Medical students, residents, registrars, fellows and specialist ICU doctors, or 'intensivists', attended the ward round, in addition to the nurse unit manager, a social worker and two physiotherapists. The ward round was directly followed by a planning meeting, where, in a room sequestered in office space away from the busyness of the ICU, the day medical team together with a social worker and nurse in charge came together to review test results and plan patient care for the day (*see* Figure 5.2).

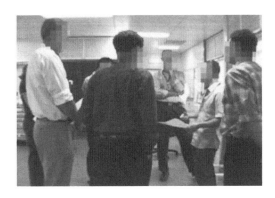

FIGURE 5.1 Intensive care unit ward round

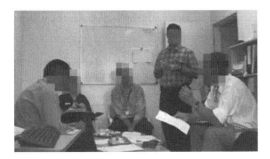

FIGURE 5.2 A planning meeting

After attending a week of such morning and evening ward rounds and the morning planning meeting, the researcher (Carroll) videoed 11 hours of ward rounds and planning meeting footage. She used a small digital handheld camera, with an additional wide-angle lens to capture large teams in small spaces, and an external directional microphone to ensure good sound quality in the busy and noisy ward environment. She also interviewed several senior doctors specifically about their views of the efficacy of the ICU's medical team communication and recorded the interviews on an audio recorder and subsequently transcribed them for analysis.

It was clear that ward round efficiency and quality was an important issue for senior doctors. 'Bernard', a senior doctor in the ICU, says this during his interview about the detail of the challenges of ward round communication:

> 'I think we could do it [ward round] a lot better, we rely on spoken communication, and if it is not effective then things get missed'. (Intensivist interview)

Junior doctors are responsible for gathering the copious details of patient status, the medical care performed, and recognising the possible future needs of each patient. This detail then needs to be structured into a narrative to be presented to the team at each ward round. Bernard highlighted the sheer complexity of grappling with large amounts of ever-changing information and ensuring its integration into patient treatment plans. This was a challenge for the senior doctors who oversee the functioning of the entire unit, yet it was even more challenging to teach the learned skill of patient trajectory planning to the junior medical staff who are still learning their craft. Bernard stated that junior staff need to learn how to convey only the important information, and to filter out detail that is not crucial for seniors to know.

> 'For the junior staff, for everyone, there is a lot of information to take in for the whole unit, the specialist covers the whole unit, there is a lot of stuff you need to be aware of, and checking, so you need to know the important things but you don't want to know the things that aren't important. That's often a bit of a problem as well'. (Intensivist interview)

The fine-detail knowledge is clearly not unimportant. Attending to the fine-detail knowledge is fundamental to patient care. Bernard carefully points out that a lack of attention to fine detail can result in aspects of care getting missed:

> 'The fine detail can get missed and if it gets busy, and if the boss doesn't look at the detail and the junior doesn't get to look at the detail or doesn't know what they are looking at little things get missed, you know [like] the central line gets left in'. (Intensivist interview)

The difficulty for the team in this ICU was finding the balance and efficiency in communicating knowledge associated with the 'big picture' patient trajectory and diagnosis (which fell primarily in the senior doctor's responsibility), and 'fine detail' patient care and test results (which was the responsibility of junior doctors). It was this tension that was explored with doctors in their video-reflexive focus group.

Exnovation in action: the video reflexive focus group

In preparation for the video-reflexive session, the researcher reviewed 11 hours of footage of ward round and planning meetings. The ICU video footage revealed a very complex flow of information between senior and junior doctors, with a lot of repetition in communication and an unclear boundary between what was discussed in the ward round and what was discussed in the planning meeting. To discuss this, all ICU medical staff were invited to a formal video-reflexive session (*see* Box 5.1).

Box 5.1 Invitation to attend video-reflexive focus group

Information notice: medical focus group

Date and time: Wednesday 26 October, 12.30 p.m.

Where: ICU meeting room

Duration: 60 minutes

Background

In April 2004, a group of three researchers . . . came and spent one continuous week observing activity in the . . . ICU. This included making video recordings of staff during their work, or in discussion of their work. The information has been analysed at an initial level and several themes will be followed through for staff input. In maintaining a grounded approach to research, staff feedback is valued and is a central focus. At this stage in the research, three focus groups will be held, one each with medical, allied health and nursing professionals. You are invited to join the medical focus group.

What is involved?

Should you decide to join the focus group, you will be shown video footage from the ward and planning rounds in the ICU. You will be invited to discuss issues raised by the video, including dealing with the tension between an abundance of detailed information and needing to know the larger main points. Secondly, the challenge of accessing and teaching 'big picture' knowledge (which is often subtle and unwritten) to junior doctors is also of interest. With your consent, this session will be videoed for confidential use by the research team. Video footage shown in these focus groups has full informed consent of those shown in the video.

> ### Voluntary participation/withdrawal of consent
>
> This study has been approved by our university's Research Ethics Committee. Participation in the study is entirely voluntary. Staff are assured of their right to refuse participation in the research programme without future repercussions at their place of employment or with any organisation involved with the research. You will be provided with both participant consent to indicate your willingness to take part, and with a revocation of consent form should you later wish to withdraw from the study. More detailed information about this study is available upon request.

To create the DVD used for the video-reflexive session, the researcher carefully selected and edited footage to show pertinent examples of senior–junior interaction and focused on the twin aims of the ward round: (1) to develop an overall impression of patient management and diagnosis and (2) to ensure sufficient attention to detail of patient care. The resulting DVD was 15 minutes in length and featured edited clips of two ward rounds, with different junior medical staff presenting to different senior medical staff who, in turn, responded to and questioned the presenting junior. The researcher needed to facilitate discussion of this footage within the framework of the larger concerns of ward round communication. Some of these concerns were reported during the interviews with senior staff, while others became evident during analysis of the video footage. To capture these issues, the researcher devised three overarching questions that were provided to the participants of the video-reflexive focus group (*see* Box 5.2).

> ### Box 5.2 The focus group guide for video-reflexivity with medical staff
>
> **Small detail, big picture: the role of the ward round and planning meeting in ICU**
>
> How do you . . .
>
> - absorb and process sufficient physiological detail without missing crucial aspects?
> - regard 'word of mouth' communication between doctors in the ward round to function in relation to the written patient notes, which are generally more widely accessible to all?
> - ensure the passage of information in both directions between the carriers of fine detail (junior staff) and the larger picture (senior staff)?

Prior to showing the DVD at the reflexive group, the researcher consulted all the medical staff featured in the edited footage and offered them a copy of the DVD that she planned to show. This gave clinicians featured in the DVD the opportunity to provide informed consent for being featured in the footage that was to be shown to the focus group. All doctors approached in this way were happy to have the DVD shown in the reflexive group 'sight unseen'.

As the examples given here reveal, it becomes clear very early in reviewing the video of real-life practices what is working and what is not. That is, there is no need to watch hours of footage. The process of watching even a few minutes of edited footage depicting a number of different instances of practice is enough to elicit plenty of comment from practitioners. Most important, the footage engenders energy and momentum for them to consider their *in situ* communication, their use of tools and technologies, and contextual features such as physical spaces. The footage moves practice out of the sphere of the taken-as-given and habituation and into a space where what happens becomes 'remarkable'. This also underlines why this process is not just 'video feedback' but 'video-reflexivity'. The point of the process is to engage practitioners in communication that goes beyond accounting for and reflecting on what happened. Instead, this communication articulates the *logic of their practice* (the totality of factors that make practice what it is) and thereby becomes capable of intervening in that logic.

On the day of the video-reflexive focus group, the researcher ensured the room was conveniently close to the ICU, large enough to accommodate a large group of doctors, and arranged with chairs in a semicircle to facilitate discussion. At the front of the room was a projector connected to a laptop computer to play the DVD. The DVD was projected onto the front wall and the sound was played through the room's audio-visual system. This set-up ensured everyone in attendance could see and hear the DVD.

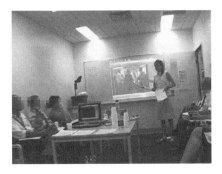

FIGURE 5.3 Researcher introducing main focuses to the video-reflexive focus group

Before showing the video footage to the 11 senior doctors in attendance, the researcher introduced the session by briefly discussing the questions (*see* Figure 5.3). Although the introductory comments provided some overall structure to the meeting, the unfolding of the meeting and the time spent on specific aspects of video footage remained in the control of the medical staff present.

The video-reflexive session lasted for 75 minutes, engaging all senior doctors in lively discussion about their approach to and enactment of ward round communication (*see* Figure 5.4). The video-reflexive session was videoed by another researcher (Rick Iedema).

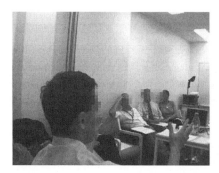 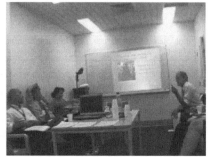

FIGURE 5.4 Lively discussion between senior intensive care doctors upon reviewing video footage

Here we list the most important discussion points emerging from the video-reflexive session.

Lack of structured communication

The most prominent issue arising from the medical reflexive session was the lack of structure in communicating both the 'big picture' patient trajectories and the significant test results and treatment detail.

> 'I ... realised there was quite a complex flow of information going on as there were several contributors about each patient but there was talking at different levels about different things, there were fragments of things that people needed to say and then the big picture about this, and then suddenly a small-detail issue ... and they leapt from one to the other and then back to the big picture. There is no build-up ... they just get thrown in as fragments from one to the other.' (Intensivist at video-reflexivity session)

Another intensivist comments on the purpose of the ward round shifting back and forth between reporting on the patient's condition and planning the patient's care.

> 'There was also the planning situation going on at the same time [as the ward round], what was happening with this patient suddenly turned into what we are going to do with the patient.' (Intensivist at video-reflexivity session)

These comments show medical staff expressing the need for a better-organised and more concise handover. The ward round was widely recognised as going on far too long, keeping doctors off the floor for longer than was needed. A structured approach seemed to be called for in order to have both adequate knowledge and time in the morning to commence patient management.

Teaching junior staff: is ward round a good time?

The footage enabled the doctors to *see* that the ward round provided only a narrow window of opportunity for dealing with a number of competing demands: gaining a full picture of patient status, negotiating management plans and/or a shared assessment of the success of pre-existing plans, and providing educative opportunities for juniors. The group readily acknowledged the importance of the ward round for providing learning opportunities to junior doctors. However, the footage alerted the senior doctors to difficulties and pressures resulting from these competing demands for juniors, particularly when they were expected to present cases.

> 'The things that I was noticing ... was this is quite daunting for the junior doctors. I realised there was a semicircle of people standing in front of them ... it looked quite an intimidating situation ... they were forced to try and create and maintain people's attention ... they had to put on an act to try and get people not to be bored. .... I hadn't realised it was an acting skill as much as a communication skill.' (Instensivist, video-reflexive focus group)

The footage made the doctors see ward round communication through the eyes of the junior doctors, which enabled them to appreciate how 'intimidating' it was for them. This raised questions about ward round effectiveness, both in terms of educational effect and in terms of the quality and safety of the care that ensues from such pressured events.

Changes made to the intensive care unit ward round

Within 2 weeks of the video-reflexivity focus group, senior medical staff had agreed upon, and implemented major changes to the way they conducted their ward round. The 14-bed ward round was split into two groups of seven patients, and an intensivist and junior doctors were assigned to each group. This meant that two ward rounds were to be run concurrently at both ends of the ICU. In addition, the planning meeting, during which the entire team met to discuss patient progress, was rescheduled to occur at midday instead of immediately following the ward round. Collectively, these two changes improved communication efficiency. They created more time for doctors to be at the patients' bedsides, during which more time was spent teaching juniors.

In addition to a change in the ward round structure and timing of the planning meeting, senior doctors devised and implemented a new documentation system. The 'ICU Daily Worksheet' was adopted to create a more structured relationship between the big-picture patient trajectory aims of the senior doctors and the detailed treatment and test results that play a big part in moving the patient towards discharge (*see* Figure 5.5).

These changes were in alignment with what the nursing staff in the ICU had been suggesting for some time in order to increase medical presence in the unit, as the nurse unit manager revealed in her interview:

> 'Since you did that with the medical staff we have had a complete turnaround with how they do the morning handover.... They get on with the day ... they see the patients. Then at twelve o'clock when they have examined the patients and seen all the things ... the patient with the X-rays, with the bloods, they come together to confirm their plan. In 1 week it is amazing. They see the X-rays in continuity with the patient, they teach while they are doing. The light globe came on. How successful was that – letting them see themselves! It's amazing. It's exactly the way that we've been asking them to look at changing. One exposure to seeing themselves'. (Nurse unit nanager, ICU)

ICU Daily Worksheet

Patient Name: _____   Date: _____

Initial as goals are reviewed: use this as basis of information to be recorded in medical file

GOAL	NOTES			
	Day	Init'l	Night	Init'l
What needs to be done for the patient to be discharged from ICU?				
Tests/procedures required				
Ventilator/pulmonary/CXR • Bundle reviewed • Strategy documented				
Sedation plan • Sedation vacation a.m. • Delirium				
Cardiovascular				
Volume status, Net goal				
Pain management				
Neuro				
GI/Nutrition/Bowel regime				
ID/Cultures/Drug levels • MRO surveillance				
Medication chart review				
Blood results				
Consultations				
CVCs, cannulas, catheters				
DVT prophylaxis	Standard Modified			
Stress ulcer prophylaxis	Standard Modified			
Mobilisation/OOB				
Skin integrity				
Family updated?				
Any social issues to address?				

FIGURE 5.5 The ICU Daily Worksheet

A senior doctor videos his own acute medical unit ward round

Would it be possible for a clinician to assume the role of the researcher described so far? Questions could be raised about the feasibility of clinicians conducting exnovation on themselves, particularly using video. Would they be able to commit enough time? Would they be able to steer clear of departmental politics? They would need to be able to inspire colleagues to sign up, engage them in discussions and reflexive sessions, record questions and answers and identify critical issues. They would also have to bring out their camera, film colleagues, edit the footage, approach colleagues for permission to use specific footage, and edit the relevant clips into a representative whole. Would an insider clinician be able to 'boundary-ride' as the researcher did in the earlier example, and assume the role of the 'clinalyst'? Gordon Caldwell's following account throws light on these and related questions.

Setting the scene

Dr Gordon Caldwell is a general physician. For a period of 12 hours every Wednesday night he is 'on take' for an acute medical unit (AMU). Being 'on take' means that all the acute general medical admissions are admitted under his name. In practical terms, this means he is accountable for their care. Yet in *actual* practice, as a senior consultant, he is only called in overnight for the more complex cases. As in the majority of UK hospitals, his team of junior doctors take histories, examine patients, make diagnoses and start treatments. However, at 8 a.m. Gordon meets with his team of junior doctors to do a 'post-take ward round' (PTWR). The purpose of the PTWR is to review the work of the night team. This team typically includes a registrar, a senior house officer, and a Year 1 doctor.

Gordon's key responsibilities include checking that his team members have the right diagnoses. He generally asks, 'Is there anything that does not "fit" with this patient?' and, 'Do the treatment plans make sense for that particular patient?' In other words, he needs to ensure that the team has thought of everything that is important. Before he goes to the patient's bedside he joins with his team for a 'pre-bedside' briefing. It is here that the night juniors narrate their account of the cases, review the blood test results, X-rays and ECGs. Gordon takes all these cases and accounts in before spending the morning communicating with patients, nurses and other health professionals at the bedside.

The method: videoing post-take round and planning meeting

Wanting to be reassured that the PTWR was effective, Gordon decided to video a typical weekend PTWR 'pre-bedside' planning meeting. For this, he used a small handheld digital camera (Flip UltraHD) and a small portable and flexible tripod (Gorillapod). This tripod meant that the video camera could be attached to almost anything – for example, a computer monitor (*see* Figure 5.6). Six days later, he reviewed the resulting footage – 90 minutes of pre-bedside ward round discussions – on his office PC at work (*see* Figure 5.7). As he went through the footage, he documented his thoughts not only about his own communication and the communication of his team, but also about the video methodology he had just started to utilise.

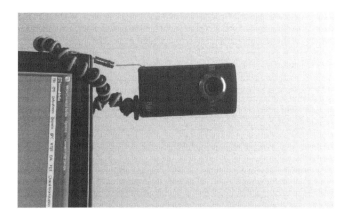

FIGURE 5.6 The Flip UltraHD and flexible tripod set-up used to video

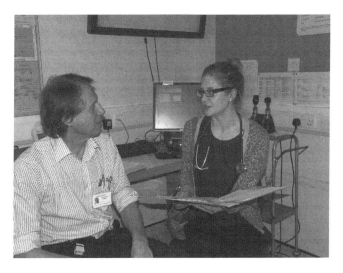

FIGURE 5.7 'Post-take ward round' communication between senior and junior doctors

Results

What observing the video footage brought home for Gordon immediately was the high number of decisions that were made in such a short time. He began to wonder whether the PTWR might well be among the most complex of human endeavours. This insight made him realise that video reveals aspects of practice that otherwise remain taken as given. For that reason alone, video is a powerful and highly productive way to reflect and learn about activities that otherwise remain taken as given, and therefore closed to reflection and intervention. It revealed the enormous achievement of the PTWR as organisational communication practice: a small group of colleagues sharing and processing so much highly complex information in such a short time.

It also became evident to him that watching yourself on video and discovering personal idiosyncrasies can be uncomfortable. Gordon himself uncovered and identified several areas of communication that he felt he needed to improve personally. Furthermore, he realised there were team processes that were in need of a change. The most obvious was that there was a lack of urgency, organisation and efficiency throughout the pre-bedside discussion phase of the PTWR, and it was this dimension that he wanted to improve most of all.

In what follows, we present the notes Gordon took from watching the PTWR video (*see* Table 5.1). He translated each of his notes into concrete learnings and, where possible, linked these to structural changes to the PTWR that have since been implemented.

TABLE 5.1 What did I learn from the 90 minutes of video that I watched?

	Observation	Example(s)	Learning	Change strategy
1	The footage revealed a lack of urgency, organisation and efficiency throughout the PTWR	(i) I witnessed myself on video having philosophical chats at several stages. (ii) There clearly were matters that could be raised later in the informal debriefing sessions over coffee.	Break the planning session into more recognisable parts.	I devised a blurb to more orderly signal the different parts of information communication in a planning session.
2	Urgency and emphasis were not always conveyed sufficiently in my voice	I realised during watching the video that by not varying my tone to emphasise important points, urgency and significance was not conveyed to team members. This was not uncommon among other contributors to the PTWR. For example, a senior house officer was discussing a woman who had deteriorated quickly, was near to death, and needed to go to the high dependency unit. Yet we discussed the case as if we were discussing the most mundane and regular of questions. The language should have been, 'Dr Caldwell, I think I need to leave the round urgently to see a lady being treated for cardiac failure and I have just received her gases showing metabolic acidosis, severe hypoxia and hypercapnia. She is full resus and escalation to ITU if needed'. Instead it took several minutes of discussion to get to the point of letting the managing doctor leave the meeting.	A change in my voice to a more direct, vigorous tone would assist in conveying the urgency of this situation and distinguishing it from other more general topics of discussion.	I will ensure I speak loudly enough.
3	We could learn to present cases more succinctly	We took so long to discuss so few patients that I believe we could learn to present patient cases more succinctly. I did point this out at one stage during the PTWR by saying, 'So to summarise what you are saying this case is . . .'. However, I do not make it plain how I want the cases presented.	With some additional attention to training, the juniors could manage to transmit as much information and thinking in under half the time, and probably even less.	(i) I devised a list of what I want to know from juniors.

(continued)

	Observation	Example(s)	Learning	Change strategy
3	(cont.)			(ii) From the list I realised I could develop an SBAR chart (Situation, Background, Assessment, Request) to be carried by juniors to help them know how to develop and report a case presentation.
4	There was no nurse	We have slipped back into just accepting that there will be no nurse present during the discussions phase. No wonder communications fail, when an essential team member is not even on the pitch. This is simply not team-working. A nurse does come in during the PTWR to get an insulin dose written up. However, I noted that I do not even challenge her and say, 'Why is there no nurse with us today?'	I have become part of the institutional indifference to lack of nurses on rounds. It is so ordinary that we do not notice it anymore. We need a senior nurse with us to contribute to, and listen to the discussions.	Speak to the head nurse to arrange for senior nursing at the start of the briefing phase to report on any urgent issues and to give a brief account of each patient.
5	The space of the briefing room is inadequate	(i) We are making so many decisions and so quickly that the room should support this process and not detract from it. The room gets too noisy and, especially on weekdays, with the door open to keep the room cool, there is a lot of noise. (ii) We all used phrases and throwaway lines that are particular to medical work. For example, 'There were several rubbish referrals from A&E', and 'Nobody died'. This is ordinary talk and would never be eliminated – it is part of the process of dealing with the frustrations that always arise. (iii) The room is too small and as a result there is not enough work surface area. The juniors are balancing notes on their knees and the others in the team need a hard surface to write request forms, CPR forms, file clerking into notes, etc.	(i) We need a quiet area for patient discussions. (ii) A passing patient might easily think we were uncaring. We need a confidential area for patient discussion. (iii) We need larger work surfaces.	We have been unable to make changes yet in relation to the 'Briefing Room'. However, this reflection resulted in my writing a 'Personal View' in the *British Medical Journal* on 'Misdiagnosis'. We are planning a rebuild of the acute medical unit and these observations will influence the layout of the Doctors' Room.

The following are examples of how Gordon sought to achieve the changes he realised were necessary upon viewing the footage. The first was to do with creating clearer signposts for the PTWR's distinct stages.

Box 5.3 Breaking up the pre-bedside briefing into recognisable chunks of information

First: This is the briefing, so let's start with introductions, then a report from the specialist registrar on how many patients need to be seen, highlight any patients that need to be seen early, and any patients needing urgent referral for tests or to other specialities.

[*dialogue of the day*]
Next: Now we move on to hear and review the cases.

[*dialogue of the day*]
Then: Now we will go out and see the cases.

The second change pertains to the specification of what Gordon wanted to know from his team members' case presentations.

Box 5.4 What I want to know from a case presentation

- Who the patient is and something to remember him/her by (e.g. 'This is a 72-year-old retired carpet fitter.')
- What the team has been treating him or her for and preferably a diagnosis (e.g. 'He has a sixth nerve palsy, and we do not know the cause.')
- The plan (e.g. 'We have done a CT brain which was clear, and we want an MRI, an ENT review, and a neurology consultation.')
- The story in slightly more detail (e.g. bring out important negatives and positives)
- Meanwhile, someone else in the team brings up test results (e.g. CT images and the blood test results on screen)
- Meanwhile, someone else starts writing the request forms (e.g. CPR form, pre-filling the TTO)

The third change Gordon was able to introduce was a clear outline for junior doctors on how to present their ward round information.

Box 5.5 Chart to assist juniors on how to present a case

Prepare
- Review patient's progress
- Read notes again
- Check all results
- ECGs, charts to hand

Patient details
- Mr Jones, 75 years
- Retired carpet fitter
- Complex case

Treating the patient for?
- Uncontrolled atrial fibrillation and cardiac failure after a recent myocardial infarction

Complicating factors?
- Chronic obstructive pulmonary disease, type 2 diabetes, lives alone

Confounding factors?
- New systolic murmur
- Pyrexia
- Anaemia, hyponatraemia

Alternative diagnoses?
- Pericarditis
- Bowel or lung neoplasm

Be ready to give further details

© Dr Gordon Caldwell, October 2010

For Gordon, having achieved these outcomes, it was evident that video reflexivity is a powerful and swift way to learn for committed professionals. He identified ways to improve communication that resulted in greater time efficiency in the hectic AMU. These changes include not only an improvement in *how* clinicians communicate during ward rounds but also the development of a number of systems that incorporated learning opportunities for junior doctors and created greater time efficiency during the PTWR. He also noted the changes that needed to be made to the physical meeting space and the equipment that it held.

Another important realisation, Gordon found, is that video reflexivity bypasses the need to set up simulations of practice. Clearly, watching footage of one's own practice can help improve professionals' everyday work, and applying this to practice generally could have a big impact on performance, safety, quality and capacity, and all without the need for major investment in developing simulation scenarios. All that is needed is a camera and some time to study the resulting footage, and edit it for reflexive feedback.

Furthermore, this approach capitalises on the active teaching that medical students and junior doctors have already received on reflection and reflexivity. Provided the observation of footage is done in a trustful group environment with someone experienced in supervision, the end result may be enhanced shared reflexivity. This is critical to countering juniors being excessively self-critical or critical of colleagues, and diminishing their confidence as a result. Viewing video footage and using it as a cue for talking about everyone's activities, decisions, thoughts and uncertainties may improve clinicians' confidence in scrutinising their own ways of working.

The biggest issue perhaps for professionals applying this approach is finding the time for the review. It took Gordon 6 days to find sufficient time to watch his footage. It is far more likely that people will find time out of work hours to review a clip, and this would require secure storage of and access to the clips by, for example, virtual private network arrangements. This is not impossible, however, since similar storage and access processes are available for educational videos.

Gordon saw a lot of opportunities for change from reviewing 90 minutes of video footage. His trial convinced him that individuals and teams could learn to improve their performance from reflection on very short clips of real perform-ance, with effects that far exceed those of content learning, formal discussion and simulated scenarios involving prefigured problem-solving.

Conclusion

The video-based research presented here took place in two modalities: (1) academic research undertaken by outside investigators and (2) practice improvement undertaken by clinicians themselves. The 'outsider' perspective of ward round communication was developed through ethnographic observations, interviews with clinical staff and video-recordings of *in situ* work. This data was subsequently analysed by the researcher, mindful of the concerns that were raised by the team's clinicians. The early interpretations and questions developed by the researcher were then placed alongside and interwoven with the clinicians' expert 'insider' knowledge during the video reflexivity session. As a result of this mutual attention to ward round communication, new knowledge and new ways of doing ward rounds were developed.

Important here is that the process itself was transparent – both for the researcher and for the clinicians. The approach to collecting, editing and showing the footage, the purpose of the focus groups and interviews, and the resulting findings and conclusions – all these developments were openly and constantly discussed between the researcher and the clinicians. The principal focus was on collaborating with the clinicians on the issues to be singled out for attention, the video clips to be used for feedback, and the conclusions to be drawn from the footage and from the subsequent discussions. Here, the researcher's principal target was not generating portable knowledge derived through applying sanctioned methods, to be published in the researcher's discipline-specific journals. Instead, the target was clinician–participant involvement in producing, selecting and making sense of the video footage, so that the clinicians and their practice benefited from the sense-making process.

When a clinician undertakes this work, they need the trust of their team. The team needs to be convinced that the point of the exercise is to learn, and not to criticise and judge. They need to know that everyone has to agree to and have a say in what gets filmed, shown back and discussed. In his account here, Gordon showed himself to be as keen to learn as he expected members of his team to be. He did not use the video to only scrutinise the performance of others. In seeking to understand his ward round, he learned about the various things that he had taken for granted, and should from now be more conscious of, or will do differently. For him, videoing practice *in situ* proved to be incredibly instructive and powerful – more so than involving his team in simulated scenarios. Video shows the mundaneness of moment-to-moment care to be hugely complex as well as harbouring critical practical effects, and it shows that practical complexity to be interpretable, workable.

Finally, both Katherine and Gordon realised that the specificity of what is in the footage fascinates rather than bores or confuses. Slips in communication, background noise, tensions between junior and senior staff, and interruptions to the ward round were deliberately not edited out of the video footage. By accommodating this complexity, exnovation homes in on actual problems using actual data. This means that the conclusions drawn and changes proposed do not need practical translation, or 'implementation' (Zuiderent-Jerak, 2007), before becoming relevant to and integrated in what people do 'normally'. This way of engendering reflexivity is not just important for preparing professionals for the *in situ* complexity they encounter at work. It is also critical for broadening the communication spectrum that binds professionals into their weave of shared practice, strengthening their capacity for distributed intelligence.

6

Introducing video-reflexivity on the ward

Some notes and observations on a Maastricht experiment

Co-authored with Twan Mulder and Corine Kooyman

Introduction

This chapter describes the experiences of a Dutch team on a neonatal intensive care unit (NICU) using video-reflexivity meetings as part of a larger project on patient safety. To introduce video-reflexivity on this ward, a social scientist (Jessica Mesman) teamed up with key clinicians: a neonatologist (Twan Mulder), the head nurse, and members of the infection control unit (Corine Kooyman). In this chapter we will describe how these clinicians made it possible to introduce video-reflexivity into the organisation, and what its outcomes were.

First, we should point out that, in this case, the reflexivity meetings were organised during the overlap of the day shift and the evening shift, during a nursing training day on infection prevention in collaboration with the infection control officer, and during a multidisciplinary training session on resuscitation led by the neonatologist. This strategy of fitting the reflexivity meetings into existing or prearranged events ensured that video-reflexivity was integrated into practice in different contexts: the swirl of activities on the ward, and a more 'peaceful and relaxed' environment of a meeting room outside the ward. Second, these different contexts brought into play various kinds of expertise, disciplinary backgrounds and levels of experience. This ensured that the participating professionals experienced video-reflexivity in different forums, each with subtly different dynamics.

The focus of the chapter will be on the common practicalities involved in preparing and executing video-reflexivity meetings. This will allow us to present some practical advice and insights. However, first we introduce the setting and the research project of which the video-reflexivity was a part. Next, we describe the practicalities involved in collecting the footage used for these meetings. Then, we discuss the reflexivity process itself.

The practical setting

The setting was the neonatology ward of a Dutch teaching hospital. The field of neonatology specialises in the care of newborn babies. The neonatology ward of this particular hospital has a tertiary care unit and as such it can provide the most advanced level of care. The NICU takes care of babies whose lives are at serious risk on account of complications linked to their delivery, congenital diseases, infections or premature birth. Because of their frail condition, these babies are highly susceptible to harm. This patient population's vulnerability calls for a high level of patient safety. Even minor incidents can result in major irreversible harm because a cascade of minor complications or small and unintended mistakes can lead to disastrous impact. For this reason, a highly supportive environment for both patients and staff is essential.

Apart from careful management of the delicate safety–efficacy balance of the medical interventions performed, the vulnerability of this patient population also calls for a strictly controlled working environment more generally. This basically means that the NICU space itself is one giant incubator – a warm, clean, carefully regulated world where overpressure and hygiene rules should ensure the lowest infection rates possible. In this environment, practice is highly structured, and professionals are highly attentive and reflexive. What might video-reflexivity add to an environment where practice is already carefully monitored, controlled and evaluated?

The research project

The research described here sought to improve understanding of the moment-to-moment unfolding of professional practice. In contrast to current patient safety research, most of which focuses on shortcomings and incidents, this project sought out highly skilled professionals and their unique expertise. In adopting this focus on the *in situ* production of safety, the project sought to confront and map the many complexities of today's health care work environment, the ways in which professionals overcome these challenges, and the resources they draw on to do so. Such an approach is important, as we still have great difficulty answering the question, 'why is health care work generally safe, despite the often limiting circumstances in which professionals find themselves?' To put this point differently: shouldn't we wonder why there are *not more* incidents, considering the high-risk environments and the innumerable complexities that define health care practices (Owen *et al.*, 2009)? Therefore, this project's focus was on how professionals produce safety, what they do to achieve this, and what video feedback might add to their safety practices.

The importance of preparatory work

In this section we discuss the preparatory activities that took place. As the field-notes cited illustrate, these activities included providing an explanation about the project, illustrating the approach by means of a DVD that exemplifies it,[15] and selecting a specific dimension of practice for the project to focus on.

> The office of the head nurse: the head nurse, one of the neonatologists, the nurse unit manager and the social researcher (Jessica) are gathered around a laptop. The researcher explains the method of video-reflexivity in detail with the help of a [HELiCS] DVD. She switches off some of the lights to ensure the screen is not over-lit. The neonatologist, the headnurse and the nurse unit manager look expectantly at the screen. The DVD together with the explanatory comments offered by the researcher make the clinicians decide to give it a 'go'. Now to avoid 'just filming anything that moves' the project has to have a focus. It is agreed that infection prevention will be the main theme of the project as it fits the researcher's focus on patient safety.

Like in the case of Katherine's ICU project discussed in Chapter 5, where clinicians' advice was sought on when and where to film, Jessica's project involved her having to acquire knowledge about procedures, protocols and medical and nursing views on infection prevention in order to determine what moments and actions to film. She consulted with several nurses, some of the neonatologists, and several members of the infection control department. Protocols relating to

---

15 In this case the HELiCS DVD (Iedema and Merrick, 2008) was used to explain and demonstrate video-reflexivity.

infection prevention were used as input as well. On the basis of this information she made a list of activities (such as hand hygiene, use of personal protective equipment), specific procedures (such as the insertion of a central catheter), and, where possible, moments during the day (right after the morning rounds) and locations in the NICU that were of importance for infection prevention. This map of the most relevant activities, their possible moments and location of occurrence, helped her to make decisions about where and when to be ready for filming.

In exploring this aspect of the research, Jessica realised that her asking questions of the clinicians revealed that they, too, were not always and necessarily able to be explicit about what was important to infection control. Her questioning therefore functioned as a kind of awareness-raising. This suggests too that if clinicians are to engage in video-reflexivity, they should take this preparatory stage seriously, and not assume that they will automatically know what is important, where important processes take place, and what to film. A thorough questioning of practice and of assumptions about it provides critical preparation for making filming and video-reflexivity choices (Carroll and Mesman, 2012).

Another critical factor is clinicians' willingness to collaborate and take the video work seriously. To achieve this, clinicians on the ward were involved in discussions about the project, and were very well informed about the purpose and process of being filmed. To inform all the relevant staff it was necessary for the researcher to be on the ward during different shifts and to present the project on a variety of occasions, such as the weekly meetings of nurses and doctors.

Besides introducing and explaining the project and its purpose, the researcher also informed clinicians about their own role and their rights. For this aim a letter was prepared – in close collaboration with the hospital's legal advisor – which stated that none of the footage would be shown to people not involved in the project or used for the purpose of performance management or individual assessment. Additionally, clinicians were informed that participation and being filmed were voluntary, and anyone could decline to be filmed at any time. This proviso is an integral part of standard ethics approvals, but it was particularly important to be emphasised in the NICU with its demanding and complex work routines. It was important to avoid anyone feeling nervous because of the presence of a camera and this resulting in a negative effect on patient safety. In the end, however, only one person (out of 105) indicated unwillingness to be filmed.

As well as the clinicians, the patients and their families have to be informed and must consent as well. In the case of an NICU, this pertains to the cohorts of parents moving through the unit. Besides explaining the project, we also asked their permission to film the doctors and nurses while they were taking care of their child. In this case we used an informed consent form that parents had to sign to give their official approval. The form also provided the opportunity for parents to withdraw after having given their approval already.

After selecting the theme (infection control), the significant actions, times and places, and informing all the relevant participants, the filming commenced.

The actual filming

The first day of filming was devoted to getting clinicians used to being filmed. There were three aspects that acted in the project's favour. First, the project was about patient safety (why things work out safely) and not about errors, so the focus was on the competencies and high quality of work processes. Second, the camera was mostly trained on what went on inside incubators. What was captured by focusing on this narrow field of activity were mostly clinicians' arms and hands, rendering much of the footage anonymous. Thirdly, the clinicians had known the researcher since the early 1990s, when she first started her research there.

When filming commenced, some clinicians were so keen to see the result that they asked to be shown the footage on the laptop immediately after filming. The researcher consented to this request, allowing the clinicians a say in the unfolding of the project, and thereby making them more comfortable with the film process, and more closely involved in the researcher's explorations and questioning.

Over a period of 3 weeks, and using a simple handheld camera, the researcher filmed all kind of activities. These activities were all related to infection prevention and ranged from entering the ward in the airlock to care activities carried out by groups of nurses. She also filmed the beginning of early morning shifts, the examination of patients by doctors and the visits of radiology department staff and other consulted specialists. She further filmed several procedures, such as the insertion of a central catheter or intravenous line from the very beginning (collecting the items needed) and up to the final acts of cleaning up in and outside the incubator and comforting the baby. Likewise, she filmed five o'clock nursing rounds as they included the replacement of lines, and the provision of food and medication, as well as less evident potential infection moments such as the morning handovers, which are done at the bedside and sometimes involve touching the patient. Another aspect of practice that was filmed pertained to forms of collaboration. Using a camera allows you to capture collaborative activity and interactive dynamics on a scale not possible with conventional ethnographic or audio-recording methods.

Practical challenges

To get a clear camera picture requires *light*. However, the NICU presented a couple of complicating factors. On this ward the patients are not in a bed but in an incubator. Some incubators are open and as such resemble a bed, which makes it easier to film what goes on. Other incubators, however, are closed boxes and this involves filming through a plastic surface. This requires much light and a clean surface, and you have to be constantly vigilant to avoid reflections off the incubator's surface. Avoiding such reflections can be problematic when the clinicians use special light sources to illuminate delicate procedures, such as a line insertion.

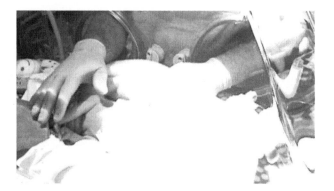

FIGURE 6.1 Reflection of light on incubator's surface

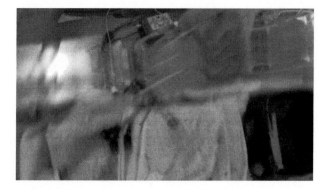

FIGURE 6.2 Distortion resulting from videoing through incubator walls

Additionally, some parts of the incubator surface are curved and as such they distort what is filmed. In practice these challenges required a 'triple focus of attention' on the part of the researcher: while filming the activities of the clinicians, she had to keep an eye on the reflecting and distorting effects of the incubator's surface, the likely filmic result produced by the camera's angle and distance, and keep in focus as well the most critical aspect that needed to be captured to adequately portray what was going on.

A second challenge is ambient *noise*. Although not all footage requires access to what is being said, in some cases good sound is essential. Yet ambient sound can be important for the clinicians who monitor ward noises for critical signals. Some noises are taken as given, as they are produced by common technologies – a heart monitor, a ventilator, a pager or a phone. Other noises are less common and more disruptive – something being dropped on the floor, a door being shut too loudly, or a conversation with high levels of emotional intensity. For the purpose of filming what goes on and picking up what is said, both too much noise and too little sound can be a problem. In the NICU, and sometimes to respect privacy, clinicians tend to speak very softly during ward rounds. Unless a directional microphone is being used, it may have trouble registering such conversation.

The third challenge is *space*. To get a good picture further requires adequate room to position oneself in order to zoom in on the activity that has to be filmed. On the NICU, the researcher filmed the activities of clinicians from different positions: one, by positioning herself at the end of the incubator in the case of two clinicians standing at each side of the incubator; another, from the side of the incubator in the case of there being only one clinician present. However, most activities on newborns are very detailed matters taking place in very small spaces. It can happen that the clinician's left hand blocks our view of what his or her right hand is doing. Or an instrument or piece of technology may obstruct our view. To find a better angle from which to film may involve moving to the other side of the bed. This takes not only time but also space – space that is not always available. It also requires great care, such as to not distract the clinicians at work. In practice it is not possible to film every action from a good angle. This can be solved through filming the same activity on different occasions.

However, sometimes interventions involve many hands and bodies. In these cases there may not be sufficient room to film the activity, except from overhead, by holding the camera high up. This researcher ended up with severe neck and shoulder problems because she didn't use a rod but, rather, held her camera above her head trying to reach over the shoulders and the heads of the clinicians in order to film what they were doing in the incubator. Sometimes she would stand like this for over half an hour or longer. Adding to the tension was the high level of concentration required while filming (zooming, avoiding reflections, selecting angles and micro-actions, etc.).

Filming clinicians at work implies non-stop *selection* about which action(s) to follow. This involves making choices not only between whether to follow a nurse or a doctor, but also between whether to capture the hand that stays in the incubator and the one that is taken out to change the settings on the respirator, as one person can execute simultaneous actions. Zooming out can partly solve this problem but this comes at the cost of missing out on other important details. In other words, filming is making choices about what activities to follow, at what level of detail, how to frame the action, where to position oneself, and when to start and when to stop filming. Filming may also be accompanied by the need to gain consent from people arriving into a scene that is in the process of being filmed. For an individual researcher this can be challenging, but a video team can solve this problem by sharing these responsibilities (Carroll and Mesman, 2012).

Selecting footage

After 3 weeks of filming various procedures, actions, moments and discussions related to infection prevention, the researcher had to categorise the footage gathered. First, all videotapes were downloaded onto the computer. Second, they were labelled with the tape's date and tape number (often more than one tape was shot on a single day). Third, each tape was carefully catalogued in terms of topic, length, actors involved and location on the tape. In this way a clear overview of the data was generated. Next, she categorised the footage into themes such as nursing rounds, intravenous line insertions, hand hygiene, doctor–nurse collaboration and medical examination. These themes were used to decide which footage would provide appropriate and sufficient information for the reflexive meetings.

In the remainder of this chapter we will focus on the different kinds of reflexivity meetings.

The weekly meetings on the ward

To organise reflexivity meetings requires insight into what might be the right time, place and pace. These may differ for every health care setting. It was decided to organise a weekly meeting on Friday afternoons between 2 and 2.30 p.m. At that time there was an overlap of the day and evening nursing shift and the doctors would be back from their lunch. In this way there was a small window of opportunity to allow some of them to sit down for half an hour and discuss their own way of working based on selected video clips. Every meeting was audiotaped by the researcher as part of her data collection.

Half an hour is not much for discussing issues in-depth, but the NICU affords little time for the clinicians to be away from their patients on top of their regular coffee and lunch breaks. However, by having the discussions in the meeting room on the ward, doctors and nurses were close to the NICU in case of an emergency. Of course, longer meetings (such as the ones Katherine was able to organise during her project, discussed in Chapter 5) would have enabled the clinicians to discuss issues in more depth, but generally such meetings may be more difficult to organise and to attract good attendance. Also, it became apparent that in a lot of instances the NICU clinicians attending the meetings discussed what they had seen in the clips over subsequent days, both with colleagues who were present and with others who had not been able to attend the meeting. The meetings were scheduled such that talk about the footage would continue from meeting to meeting, with every subsequent meeting providing new food for thought. In this way continuity was created across the meetings, and the reflexive effect of the project was enhanced.

On the NICU the weekly video-feedback sessions initially produced the same response elicited during the first days of filming: people giggling when being filmed or when seeing themselves or a colleague on the screen. However, it would only take minutes before people felt more at ease and started to concentrate on what went on. In cases where one of the attending staff members played a major role in the selected footage they were contacted about this beforehand to ask their permission for the clip to be shown. This ensured that they did not find themselves suddenly and unexpectedly the centre of everyone's attention, and had the opportunity to refuse the clip being shown.

Facilitating the reflexive sessions, the researcher had to remain sensitive to the responses from the group attending the reflexive session. The importance of this was borne out by a clip that elicited much critical comment from the nurses. Before showing this clip, the researcher played another one showing how a nurse carefully swaddles a severely premature baby into a cloth so as to support and comfort the baby:

> The baby in the incubator is hooked up to many lines and tubes and the nurse asks for help. Someone arrives. Now four hands take care of the baby. The soft cloth is carefully wrapped and folded around the baby very slowly to avoid the baby experiencing stress. After some time they are done. The baby is perfectly swaddled, and is soon sound asleep.

The video clip of this event revealed a perfect execution of what was a new procedure. Everyone watching was impressed. Another example showed the same seamless orchestration of actions. Again everyone in the room was impressed.

The members of the 'comfort team'[16] who were present seemed stunned. One of them said, 'I cannot believe what I have just seen! My impression was that hardly anyone used our technique, and that it was hardly implemented. I am so happy with what I have just seen.' Then those present started to make guesses about whose skilful hands they had just witnessed. It turned out to be those of a nurse and a doctor. One nurse suggested the doctor was probably helpful because of the presence of the camera. To the relief of everyone in the room, the other nurses corrected her immediately, dispersing the tension.

Showing this footage made it possible to evaluate a comfort technique that was only recently introduced. During the discussion, not only the prevailing perception about the technique hardly having been implemented could be corrected but also views about the modality of collaboration between nurses and doctors could be reassessed. Having achieved a lot of positive comment from the group, the researcher chose to play a clip rather different to the ones just discussed:

> Four hands carefully enfold a baby in a cloth. While one hand holds an intravenous line in the air, two other hands slowly move the cloth underneath. The hands move slowly and we can hear two people speaking softly. At the very end of the procedure the four hands rest beside the now fully covered baby. It seems the two clinicians take a moment to enjoy the result of their action. Suddenly we can hear footsteps coming near. Now the camera zooms out and focuses on a nurse next to the incubator. The footsteps stop as one of the doctors steps into the frame and asks: 'can you please unwrap the baby for me because I want to examine him'. The camera zooms in on the face of the nurse, who looks perplexed.

The video ends. This time no introductory comments of the researcher were needed as the nurses in the room immediately started to howl: 'unbelievable', 'this has happened to me many times', how frustrating', and so forth. The doctors present quickly responded to this outburst:

> 'Indeed, very frustrating and not just for you, but also for us. We too do not want this to happen and feel more than uncomfortable to ask you this. But we have to work out the details of our examination in this room and we have no idea when you do what.'

---

16 These are made up of clinicians specialised in comfort techniques and in introducing new ways of working on the ward.

The group dynamics were positive enough for them to confront a shared frustration, and this enabled them to start looking for a solution.

As Jessica's project was about the weave of safety instead of the causes of errors and incidents, the reflexivity meetings always started with a focus on successful practice: 'what went well and why?' For one, this enabled the clinicians to see that their own activities closely conformed to the unit's protocols. Even more important, they were alerted to how different clinicians performed the same protocols in different but legitimate ways. This alerted them to the various gradations of safety and practical skill that are embedded in what they do. By watching each other perform highly skilled and carefully proceduralised activities, they were enabled to learn and expand their own ways of working.

There were also less predictable responses to such footage. On one occasion, clinicians expressed surprise about the size of their hands compared with the tininess of their patients. In practice they never look at their own hands in this way, as their focus is on what they are doing. This too made them marvel at their own achievements. On another occasion, they expressed pride about how precise, accurate and seamless their team collaborations were, and how well they carried out complex procedures. They also seemed proud of more mundane – yet very important – things, such as how clean everyone's nails were.

However, regardless of the initial focus on safe and sound ways of working, in every reflexivity meeting mistakes, errors and problems were also part of the discussion. It did appear as if people felt more at ease discussing problems than their own successes, skills and competencies. In some cases the discussion targeted clinicians who performed tasks in ways that were considered to be sub-ideal, or even substandard. For example, one of the clips showed colleagues enacting outdated ways of working. The ensuing discussion was about how difficult it was to get the message through about practice change, and about the difficulties of communicating such changes to a nursing workforce of more than 80 people, many of whom work part-time.

On another occasion, the nurses present corrected a resident who was shown to enact a procedure incorrectly. On yet another occasion, a clip showed how the neonatologist and a nurse performed a perfect sterile insertion of a central catheter despite being interrupted by colleagues who asked all sorts of questions about the condition of other patients. Several critical remarks were made in response to these clips, and directed at the people responsible. However, the trust that was engendered through first focusing on the team's achievements may have prevented the discussion from descending into conflict, and helped maintain the group's focus on shared learning.

Learning about learning: video-reflexivity as pedagogic acceleration

Now looking back we can conclude that video-reflexivity as a teaching instrument has many advantages over the more traditional forms of teaching, whether those involving the transfer of content knowledge, problem-based learning or even scenario-based simulation. In the following interview extract, the infection control officer reflects on her experience of a nursing training day and captures well the various advantages of using video clips for learning:

> 'An important aspect is that nurses can discuss their own work among themselves. It is a discussion among equal professionals instead of a doctor who – with all best intentions – presents a lecture about infection prevention. In the video-reflexivity meeting nurses were among themselves and felt at ease to discuss their own and each other's ways of working.
>
> An additional advantage of video is that it provides 'evidence'. Everyone can see how things are done, so there is no discussion about whether these situations did occur or not. With the video clips we have proof, so to speak. Now discussions did not dwell on whether these kinds of situations actually happen on their ward or not. Instead it was about possible ways of improvement. So it saves time as they focus immediately on potential solutions.
>
> A very simple advantage, of course, is that you can stop the tape whenever you want to. You can also use the same footage for different purposes. Different questions can be asked on the basis of the same video clip.
>
> Images make a stronger impression than numbers. Moreover, they [clinicians] recognise themselves on the screen. This makes it more interesting and in this way you capture their full attention, which in turn makes it easier for them to remember what has been discussed.
>
> Watching each other's actions on a video makes it not only more interesting, it also underlines that we discuss their ways of working [in specific] and not infection prevention in general. They are much more involved [in that way].'

Another important aspect of video-reflexivity is the involvement and commitment of senior staff. Their involvement means they have the courage and generosity to be vulnerable in front of colleagues. In doing so, they demonstrate that shared discussions about one's way of working offer learning opportunities rather than being considered as a potential threat or a criticism. Showing footage that features senior staff who are willing to scrutinise their ways of working, and consider the possibility of improving what they do is an important aspect of creating a safe atmosphere and commitment to learning.

According to the infection control officer, there are other advantages as well:

> 'Another advantage of using video over PowerPoint presentations is that people can see where they do their work. Their equipment, materials and workbenches are all clearly visible. They do not only recognise their own work setting, but look at it from a different angle. In this way they observe how they use the space of the ward. They identify, for example, incongruous aspects of the spatial design of the ward, like a trash bin close to the place where they prepare the medication. Or they notice how some parts of the ward are ordered in an impractical way. During the video meeting we showed them the preparation of an IV-line. Because they know the place they were able to assess to what extent this area was indeed the right place to do that preparation.'

Finally, video-reflexivity provides critical input for the clinicians and for the infection control officers about how to limit cross-infection. In their reflexive discussions, the clinicians were enabled to reason about and compare their approaches to infection prevention. The infection control officer, again:

> 'What I like very much is that the footage also shows clearly how well they do certain things. I was really impressed by how good a team they are. These are issues we hardly discuss within the standard format of training. There it is all about prevention, potential dangers and possible mistakes. Video is so much more positive. You see the things going well … In this way you can also consider video-reflexivity as a positive contribution to your immediate tasks.'

Conclusion

Video-reflexivity is a complex process, much like clinical care itself. It poses many uncertainties for the researcher, and for the clinicians who participate in it. The researcher needs to make clinicians comfortable with what is still an unusual approach: to film practices that many still consider as being off-limits for outsiders. The researcher is burdened with winning professionals over and persuading them of the usefulness of being filmed and of reflecting on the resulting footage.

The feedback sessions can also be unpredictable, with some discussions being surprisingly productive, and others becoming quite political, defensive and even conflictual. Many comments were *emotional* responses. Viewing footage clearly alerts those present to the *felt* dimensions of their work, and this puts at risk the *relational* dimensions of that work. These responses may be confirming, but can also at times be challenging.

We believe that the productive impact of video reflexivity emerges from people's emotional engagement with the footage. Of course, the emotional dimensions of video reflexivity need to be managed by the person initiating this work, and this calls for excellent facilitation skills. But, as we know from Dewey's work, emotion, or what he called *impulse*, is critical to enabling and ensuring learning (Dewey, 1922). Without emotional involvement, practitioners are much less likely to benefit from reflexive sessions. Emotion connects them to one another, and it reinforces an immediacy of insight. Learning without emotion is little more than remembering. When emotion is put into play, learning comes into its own because emotion is 'an agent of steady reorganization of custom and institutions' (Dewey, 1922: 72).

> Impulses are the pivots upon which the reorganization of activities turn, they are the agencies of deviation, for giving new directions to old habits and changing their quality. (Dewey, 1922: 67)

Many instances are now available of clinical teams having used video to intervene in their clinical handover processes (Broekhuis and Veldkamp, 2007; Iedema *et al.*, 2009d), their ward rounds (Carroll *et al.*, 2008) and their infection control practices (Iedema and Rhodes, 2010). However, measurement of the impact of these improvements on clinical outcomes is as yet some time off. Overall and anecdotally, the effects of video-reflexivity on team communication are significant, and the practice of using video to enhance care is spreading not just in clinician training but also among more senior front-line professionals (Kaiser Permanente, 2010).

These developments support the view that video is an important enabler. Video may open the world of care up to professionals who, by dint of being ensconced in care environments their whole career, have un-learned to be surprised about what they do. They have forgotten how to observe their own ways of working as outsider patients do, or in the case of the NICU, as parents do. Their long working hours, coupled with the often frantic pace of the care provided to rising numbers of increasingly complex patients, prevent professionals from taking time out to reflect on the effects and effectiveness of their work.[17] In that regard, video reflexivity offers a fast and incisive countermeasure. The potential of video for accomplishing rapid practice reform is further exemplified by what we discuss in the next chapter: the institutionalisation of a handover protocol at the ambulance–emergency department interface.

---

17 We note that practitioners are able to 'difficilitate' (rather than 'facilitate') the video reflexivity meetings. The experiences of Gordon Caldwell as described in the previous chapter affirm this. Also, Jessica Mesman has successfully trained NICU clinicians to do their own filming, editing footage and chairing the reflexivity meetings. The NICU has since adopted clinician-driven video-reflexivity as integral to their own professional development and practice improvement.

7

Improving post-operative handovers using video-reflexivity

The Utrecht experience

Co-authored with Elizabeth van Rensen,
Bas de Vries and Cor Kalkman

Introduction

This chapter describes the experiences of the team at the University Medical Center Utrecht. They ran a video-based exnovation project in the Netherlands involving several local hospitals. With Professor Cor Kalkman as principal investigator, and Elizabeth van Rensen and Bas de Vries as researcher-facilitators, the project engaged six hospitals to participate in videoing post-operative handovers, and play the footage back to staff involved in the handovers. The project achieved remarkable changes and improvements within a relatively short time. This chapter records and reflects on the reflexive process and its accomplishments.

From a traditional to an exnovating approach to improving handovers

Effective communication between health care providers is essential for safe care. A breakdown in communication may contribute to serious incidents. A critical communication event is the clinical handover (World Health Organization and Joint Commission International, 2007). It is now evident that inadequate clinical handover communication poses a major risk in health care (Solet *et al.*, 2005). Inadequate handovers lead to information loss and thereby endanger the continuity and safety of care (Arora *et al.*, 2005). Improving handovers is therefore an important goal for patient safety (US Joint Commission, 2012).

For the purpose of the Utrecht project, clinical handover was defined as 'the transfer of professional responsibility and accountability for some or all aspects of care for a patient or group of patients, to another person or professional group on a temporary or permanent basis' (World Health Organization, 2008). The focus of the project was on post-operative handovers. Post-operative handovers occur when a patient is transferred from the operating room to the recovery room or intensive care unit (ICU). These handovers cover the needs and progress of unstable patients straight after their operation. There may be time pressure on those delivering the handover, as the anaesthesia team needs to start the next operation with minimal turnover time. Furthermore, post-operative handovers often include, besides the transfer of information and responsibility, the handing over of monitoring equipment, requiring clinicians to connect the electrocardiogram or ECG, calibrate the arterial lines, and reconnect the ventilator and the transfer infusion pumps.

In this technological environment, it is imperative that the 'recovery' nurses (those receiving the patient after their operation) appropriately reconnect the various types of equipment. This means there will be considerable attention on the technological aspects of the handover. While critical, this technology focus may distract from listening carefully to the verbal handover, particularly when this is communicated concurrently. Indeed, qualitative studies have found that handovers in the post-anaesthesia care unit were characterised as being event-driven, time-pressured, prone to competing demands on people's attention and causing distractions and often subject to incomplete information transfer (Nagpal *et al.*, 2010; Smith *et al.*, 2008). Aiming to address these tensions and demands, the 'Patient Veiligheid Centrum' (Patient Safety Centre) at the Utrecht University Medical Centre in the Netherlands set up a large multicentre project to improve post-operative handovers across a number of participating hospitals.

The project was initially structured to be a prospective, controlled (before–after) intervention study. The primary aim was to develop and implement a structural, standardised handover procedure in all participating centres. The original study design started with a pre-intervention period that included a study into factors that influence communication during handover situations. The plan was to develop a standardised handover procedure. During the intervention period, the plan was that this standardised handover procedure be implemented in all participating centres. To determine the impact of the intervention on the quality of handovers, actual handovers were going to be videotaped by a professional cameraman. It was intended that these videotapes were going to be analysed by researchers using a standardised coding scheme to support the development of the handover protocol.

The development of the ideal standardised handover protocol turned out to be a challenge. A steering committee, including key persons of the participating centres, was unable to reach agreement on the content of the standardised protocol. Discussions stagnated on the definition of a structured handover. Interestingly, it was a little easier for professionals to determine *what* should be spoken about during a handover than to reach agreement on *how* a handover should be performed. However, overall the large diversity of local circumstances made it impossible for the committee to articulate and agree on a single standardised handover procedure. As deliberations progressed, the steering committee key persons realised that health care provision is too complex and settings too varied to allow a single handover protocol across sites, even in a domain as well circumscribed as post-operative handover.

At the same time, what inspired these discussions was the richness of the real-life videotaped handovers that were shown as examples of what was videoed. People realised it was extremely valuable to view this material, because it revealed aspects of practice to which they had never paid attention. When Professor Cor Kalkman heard Rick Iedema speak at the Isala Clinic in Twente (east Netherlands) in 2008, Cor proposed to introduce video-reflexivity to the Utrecht project as a way to resolve the dilemma. The project team agreed to trial the method.

Applying the video-reflexive method radically changed the project's approach to improving handovers. The most significant changes were the following. First, showing the footage of videoed handovers back to the clinicians involved was now the intervention – not imposing a formalised protocol on those clinicians designed by a committee of experts from elsewhere. Instead of the researchers and committee members determining how handover should be done, clinicians in the local sites viewed footage of their actual, *in situ* practices, discussed the implications of what they saw, and collectively worked out what they could do to rationalise the handover process. The video footage no longer acted as merely an 'objective record' of handover communication for researchers to analyse against generalised criteria. Now, the video footage was used to inspire discussion among front-line clinicians themselves about their own local practices, their own problems, and the opportunities and potentials embedded in those practices.

Second, not the researchers nor the committee but the clinicians in the participating hospitals became the judge of what worked and what did not work in their own practices. Here, attention was paid not just to what people talked about, but also to how (and when) they manipulated technologies and other resources (e.g. beds). Viewing of the footage and multidisciplinary discussion enabled the clinicians to critique their own handovers on a range of dimensions and propose relevant changes. This led to the participating teams devising their own solutions and changes, each with varying levels of effectiveness, but each tailored to suit their specific site's location, spaces and technologies.

Importantly, across the participating hospitals, the solutions and changes proposed were not just site-specific but also had elements in common. We touch on these commonalities in the chapter's concluding discussion. What this suggests however is that allowing practitioners to develop their own local solutions may lead them to arrive at compatible if not similar solutions.

Third, because the clinicians had now taken over the role of judges and designers, they were also better positioned to take on the role of 'implementers'. Having seen themselves on screen, they were now keenly aware of the potential embedded in and problems affecting their own ways of working. The footage had shown them the effects of how they as teams had become habituated into taking specific ways of doing handovers for granted. This enabled them to target in a very precise way the times, resources, places and people needing to be targeted to effect a change.

Finally, seeing themselves on screen and devising new ways of doing handover gave participating clinicians insight into the power of reflexive learning in and for practice (Iedema, 2011). For many of the participating clinicians, it was not so much the new handover solution as the transformative experience of reflecting on practice that produced new insights into work organisation. This realisation is likely the most powerful of video-reflexivity: front-line staff being enabled to effectively and efficiently produce solutions that readily fit in with their existing weave of practices, people, technologies and spaces (Bate, 2000). This comes about when practitioners see that what they do and say is not 'natural and necessary', but that things can be different and are open to change (Iedema *et al.*, 2009e).

Ultimately, six hospitals agreed to adopt the new video-reflexive approach. In adopting the video-reflexive approach, they preferred new footage to be shot rather than using footage from the previous incarnation of the project. This was perhaps because now they realised they were going to be more closely involved in the shooting, selecting of clips, scrutinising and problem-solving. In the next part of this chapter, we will first describe our interactions with the hospitals and the structured method that we were able to develop as the project unfolded. Next, we will provide a narrative description of specific achievements at each hospital. Finally, we will present our conclusions and some questions remaining with regard to using video-reflexivity as a structured tool for improving complex processes in health care.

Video-reflexivity: a structured method to improve complex processes in health care

By and large, the Utrecht project drew on HELiCS, a video-reflexive ethnography improvement kit developed at the Centre for Health Communication, the University of Technology, Sydney, as part of the Australian Clinical Handover Initiative Project (Iedema and Merrick, 2008; Iedema *et al.*, 2009d). The HELiCS resource was funded by the Australian Commission on Safety and Quality in Health Care. HELiCS is an acronym for 'Handover: Enabling Learning in Communication for Safety'. It was Rick Iedema's 2009 HELiCS presentation in Twente that caught Cor Kalkman's interest.

HELiCS prescribed a number of stages for the deployment of video in health care settings. The original stages defining HELiCS were slightly adapted to suit Dutch needs, resulting in the following five-step method (*see* Table 7.1).

The basic principle here is that front-line clinicians gain a say in what aspects of their work are to be captured, how the resulting footage is to be edited and what is to be shown back to them. They are clear that they are in charge of formulating conclusions from what they see and using those conclusions to redesign what they do and say. The power of the visual medium is that these deliberations will not be constrained by a narrow analytical focus on 'what do people convey as part of the handover and in what order'. Instead, deliberations can touch on what is said, who says them, when these things are said, how the saying interweaves with moving and reconnecting the various kinds of technological equipment,

TABLE 7.1 Stages for the deployment of video in health care settings

Step	Description
1: Engaging management and familiarising front-line staff with the video method	It is critical to obtain management support for the method. While this will not guarantee front-line clinician support, it promotes faith in the positive impact of the method and reassures staff that the risk of capturing potentially subpoenable material is outweighed by the advantage of team learning. As for front-line staff, facilitators will need to work on developing trust relationships with those clinicians who are willing to participate in the videoing. Trust is engendered by facilitators spending time on the wards or in the relevant departments as non-participant observers, before bringing along their video cameras. Also, a series of meetings needs to be arranged with front-line staff, to explore their understandings of the video method, their responsibilities when signing up, ground rules (about ending one's relationship with the project or questioning the videoing of specific events), and practical issues that they find worthy of being videoed.
2: Videotaping and 'hot feedback'	Handover events are videotaped over a set period of between a few days and a couple of weeks (depending on resources available). On the day of videoing and once the videoing has concluded, sections of the videos can be immediately shown back to individual professionals (one-on-one). This hot-feedback component signals to clinical professionals that the facilitator-researchers value their input, and that they have a role to play in deciding what is valuable footage and what is not, and it enables facilitators to gain initial insight into prominent issues in the footage, relevant foci for improvement, as well as sensitive matters (pertaining to specific individuals or actions visible in the footage and which may be detrimental if shown publicly). Hot feedback also offers the facilitator-researchers the opportunity to ask for permission to show the recordings to others. In doing this, facilitators are enabled to fine-tune their videoing, building confidence they are videoing the right thing, that the participating professionals are happy with what is going on, and that they are capturing useful data. The facilitators stop with videoing when time runs out (and not much footage is needed to have a good reflexive session!), or when saturation is reached (no new issues are captured). Depending on the level of detail required, and depending on the degree of familiarity on the part of the researcher with the site and the practice, saturation tends to set in anywhere between 1 and 3 weeks, but this is a rough guide only. At the end of step 2, many if not most professionals have seen some footage, feel comfortable with the process and may have ideas for improvement.

Step	Description
3: Selecting and editing video fragments	Based on the input of the professionals and the facilitators' own expertise, the facilitators make compilations of video clips that capture the discussion themes and/or specific issues, problems or successes. Clips used for feedback should not be more than 2–4 minutes long. Before being shown in public, clip selections should be tested one-on-one with on-site champions to ensure no sensitive actions or behaviours are shown and no relationships are damaged. Facilitators have to have a bank of clips and work out how to structure the discussion; that is, they need to be clear about the questions and issues they would like to see raised, even if the resulting deliberations end up moving in very different directions.
4: Multidisciplinary feedback	The selected clips are presented at (ideally, multidisciplinary) feedback sessions. The facilitators may structure their presentation on the basis of what they have videoed and heard during previous meetings and fast-feedback. The feedback meeting may be videoed to capture the groups' responses and creative thinking. Frequently, the discussion will flow quite freely and will touch on a great variety of topics. Here, facilitation comes into its own; the facilitators need to skilfully guide the participants to address matters that matter and that can be feasibly changed. In many instances too, groups will steer the discussion towards important issues and useful outcomes. Ideally, the meeting concludes with an agreement on a change, and identification of a person responsible for overseeing the change and its communication to staff, and a starting date.
5: Recording the change	When the change that was devised during the feedback meeting or meetings (e.g. a new handover format, or a handover form, or a checklist) is put into practice, it is important that this change and the new practices buttressing it are videoed. Time needs to be allowed of course for the practice to 'gain traction'. A date is agreed when the teams are ready to be videoed enacting the change. A further set of feedback meetings or evaluations can be initiated with the purpose of engendering conviction among staff that they are capable of 'continuous improvement'.

where the saying occurs in the space available, how non-verbal kinds of communication can be made to play a role, and so forth. The reports from the participating hospitals confirm that people's discussions and proposed solutions were at once broad-ranging and specific to accommodate the different sites' unique locale, patients, professional skill-mix and technologies.

Video-reflexive exnovation in action: tales from six hospitals
· · · · · · · · · · · · · ·

Teams made up of front-line clinician volunteers from six different hospitals adopted video-reflexivity to improve their handovers. In this section we present their case studies. In four hospitals, the focus was on handovers from the operating theatre to the recovery room; in one hospital, the focus was on handovers after cardiothoracic surgery at a paediatric ICU, and the last hospital focused on handovers following cardiothoracic surgery at an adult ICU.

Hospital 1: Post-operative handover improvement

Hospital 1 is a large teaching hospital with 889 beds and more than 3500 employees. This hospital focused on post-operative handovers at recovery. In this hospital, post-operative handovers are performed using a special post-operative form. This form is being updated each year to make sure that its users (surgeons, recovery room nurses, anaesthetic nurses and anaesthesiologists) have an opportunity to specify their post-operative handover expectations. The last update of the form involved some changes in its structure and an expansion of the section on surgical information. The recovery nurses were very satisfied that the handovers were adequate because the clinicians relied on the form for their handover. The surgeons were hardly ever present during the handover, but the form was understood as sufficient for rendering their handover information available.

The recovery room nurses also knew however that the form could pose problems. The anaesthesiologists often ticked the box 'pain medication and fluids according to protocol'. However, this was often done for convenience sake, leaving the recovery room clinicians at times unclear about exactly what medication was administered.

Viewing the footage intervened in this situation in important ways. First, the anaesthesiologists realised that their use of the form posed a risk, and that it was essential that the form be filled in completely and correctly. Second, the footage made the recovery room nurses and the anaesthesiologists aware of the discrepancies between their verbal handover and the structure of the form. They recognised that if the verbal handovers followed the order of the items on the form, they might be more predictably structured and therefore less likely cause confusion. Third, they agreed that there was an item still missing on the form: the emotional state of the patient before receiving anaesthetics. For the recovery room nurses, this information can be helpful for when the patient wakes up. This information was added to the form.

Finally, viewing the footage alerted the clinicians to another important issue: how does the handover ensure the privacy of patients? The footage revealed that the recovery nurses did not always close the curtains when examining a patient. This privacy concern was exacerbated by something else that the footage revealed: the considerable number of relatives allowed into the recovery room, a practice that had become more and more accepted over time. Originally, relatives were allowed in to benefit the patients. On viewing the footage however, the recovery room nurses became conscious of how large numbers of relatives could inconvenience other patients. Importantly, their presence was also realised to be disruptive to their own handover practice. In these ways, the footage raised clinicians' awareness of the vulnerability both of patients and of the recovery room handover process, and it enabled them to introduce a range of changes making their work and their patients safer.

Hospital 2: Post-operative handover improvement

Hospital 2 is a large teaching hospital with 1085 beds and more than 3600 employees. Here, the focus was also on post-operative handovers at the recovery room. Even before the video project commenced, the recovery room nurses were very critical of the way post-operative handovers were carried out at recovery. They felt they were often not given adequate and sufficient information. In their view, the anaesthesiologists and the surgical nurses cut corners when it came to giving handovers, wanting to return to the operating room as quickly as possible and get on with the next operation. During pre-video discussions, the recovery room nurses mentioned that questions often came up after the anaesthesiologist had already left the recovery room. They then had to phone the anaesthesiologist for additional information.

On viewing the footage, however, the recovery room nurses realised that they were not really listening to the verbal handovers. One person admitted, 'I pretend to listen to what you are saying, but in reality I don't hear it. I obviously think to myself, I will look it up later'. Upon seeing this, both the anaesthesiologists and the recovery room nurses agreed that the handovers at the recovery room had to be redesigned. First, the handovers had to be more efficient. They agreed that the responsible recovery room nurse should be able to focus on what is being said without being distracted. This meant that during the verbal information transfer she should not be busy with the patient. The patient should be hooked up to the monitoring equipment before the verbal handover starts.

A second change was that the content of the verbal handover was given a clearer structure. This is because, upon seeing themselves on video, staff experienced their handovers as chaotic. Relevant information was not being transferred while other items were mentioned repeatedly during one handover. It was common for the handover giver to finish and then after a while remember something else that needed to be conveyed, and reinitiate the handover. The recovery room nurses recognised that it was difficult for those listening to recall what was being said under these circumstances. They agreed that the different topics of a verbal handover had to be in an agreed order. Furthermore, mentioning irrelevant information and repeating information had to be reduced to a minimum.

A third change was the implementation of a formal conclusion to the handover with a clearly identified opportunity for questions. This signalled to all present that now the handover was over, and that, if there were no further questions, new tasks could be initiated. To implement these improvements an acronym was invented: PIRAMIDE. This stands for Patient connected (to machines), Identification of patient and patient record, Relevant medical history and allergies, Anaesthetic technique used and type of operation, Medical details, Instructions filled, Clear handover? and End of handover.

Interestingly, at the same time an electronic patient data management system was being implemented at the hospital's operating theatre. This system included a time-out procedure that had to be executed during all steps of the operating process. PIRAMIDE was included in this patient data management system where PIRAMIDE became the post-operative step of the time-out procedure. This resulted in the redesigned handover procedure being very easily implemented, as it fitted perfectly within the new system.

Hospital 3: Improving post-operative handover

Hospital 3 is a small community hospital with 494 beds and more the 2100 employees. This hospital performs about 15 000 operations yearly. In this hospital, the participating research team also focused on post-operative handovers in the recovery theatre. During the focus groups and interviews, the anaesthetic nurses and the recovery room nurses both acknowledged that there was much variation in the way the post-operative handovers were performed. The structure and content of these handovers were understood to be dependent on the persons involved and on the context where the handover was given. Some people were known to provide a lot of information while others provided only the minimum. The transfer of monitoring equipment and the transfer of verbal information often occurred simultaneously, creating a very busy handover process. If the recovery room nurse was still busy with another patient, the anaesthetic nurse would connect the patient up and the verbal handover would start when the recovery room nurse finally arrived. All this meant that the post-operative handover suffered from a lot of unpredictability.

Video footage of this site's handovers confirmed there was quite some variation in how the handovers were delivered to recovery room staff. A prominent problem arose from the recovery room clinicians trying to reconnect the patient to the technology and the theatre clinicians communicating the handover at the same time. The reconnection process involved much noise and movement and this made it near impossible to hear the information that was being provided.

When viewing the footage, both the theatre clinicians and the recovery staff realised that it was critical to first reconnect the patient and then start the verbal handover. However, a few people were concerned that this might take more time and this was not always possible. On the other hand, most people acknowledged that the handovers *during* which patients were reconnected were quite chaotic. They also realised that connecting the equipment and communicating the handover at the same time meant that people were less able to have eye contact. Lack of eye contact was experienced to be a key cause of the handover coming across as unpredictable and unstructured. The staff concluded that the importance of separating the transfer of monitoring equipment from the transfer of information outweighed the risk of the handover taking slightly more time.

Another issue that arose was that in some cases there were two recovery room nurses present at the bedside during a handover. On viewing the footage the anaesthetic nurses recognised that it was not always clear to them who was the responsible recovery room nurse who should receive the handover. They realised that it was essential to identify the responsible recovery room nurse before starting the verbal handover. To achieve this, staff agreed to standardise the post-operative handovers by implementing a five-step handover process: (1) anaesthetic nurse and recovery room nurse reconnect the patient to the monitoring equipment together; (2) the anaesthetic nurse asks, 'Can I start with the verbal handover?'; (3) the anaesthetic nurse transfers information to the responsible recovery room nurse; (4) there is a standard order of items mentioned during the verbal handover – name patient, type of operation, type of anaesthesiology, specific details, post-operative policy, and (5) the anaesthetics nurse asks before leaving, 'are there any questions?'

Four months after the conclusion of the project, Elizabeth and Bas interviewed clinicians originally involved in the project at this site. A team leader commented:

'Normally health care improvements are invented behind a desk, written on paper and dropped on those on the work floor with little notice. And then we are surprised that it doesn't work. Well, I became enthusiastic [about video-reflexivity] because of the different way in which it frames improvement and how it approaches a problem. First, we visualise what the problem is ... by using footage. After viewing and discussing the footage together ... in a plenary session we decide how we can improve [practice]'.

An anaesthetic nurse who they interviewed commented:

'The footage is very confronting. You do the best you can, but there are always things that can be improved. I saw this so clearly in the footage showing myself talking to a colleague. It was very informative. You think that you can do a quick handover if you start talking while the patient is still being connected, but then it (the information) does not get through to the recovery room clinicians'.

Hospital 4: Post-operative handover improvement

Hospital 4 is an academic hospital that performs about 23 000 operations each year. As did the teams discussed above, this hospital's team also focused on post-operative handovers in the recovery room. The pre-video-reflexivity discussions confirmed the clinicians' shared concerns about the efficacy of their handover communication processes.

On viewing the footage produced by the hospital's own research team, the anaesthesiologists and the recovery nurses agreed that their handovers were very complex and warranted being streamlined. The footage showed that the transfer of verbal information and connecting the patient to the monitoring equipment was done simultaneously most of the time. The footage also made the clinicians aware that some handover information was provided twice, while other information was not mentioned at all. They further realised that there was no eye contact between the handover giver and the receiver of the information, particularly when the transfer of monitoring equipment and the transfer of information was done simultaneously. It was agreed that the lack of eye contact made it impossible to check whether the receiver had understood or even heard the information handed over, or whether they had questions.

Having had their concerns about the complexity of their handovers confirmed when videoing the footage, the anaesthesiologists and the recovery nurses decided to change how they structured their post-operative handovers. The most important change they agreed on was to isolate the doings from the sayings.

Thus, they decided to first reconnect the patient to the monitoring equipment and then, when that was done, start with the verbal information transfer. For its part, the verbal transfer was subjected to a more structured approach as well. An order of handover information delivery was agreed on and a form was designed to guide the handover.

One year after implementation of this new handover practice, Elizabeth and Bas again videoed a number of handovers. After viewing this footage, all participants observed the enormous difference between the previous and the more recent, redesigned handover practice. The more recent footage showed that separating the transfer of equipment and the transfer of information had now become common practice. The clinicians also noticed that the transfer of verbal information was more structured and much clearer. In addition, everyone acknowledged that the recovery room had become a quieter place. They agreed that the standardised order in which items of the verbal information were presented was preferable to the original free-delivery approach. However, the new handover form was subsequently found not to be useful. Instead, staff decided to adopt an already existing checklist in use in the operating theatre. This checklist had been used to help theatre clinicians prepare for their post-operative handover, and it was agreed that it would be useful for addressing the needs of the recovery room clinicians as well.

After viewing the old and new footage, one recovery nurse commented:

> 'I was surprised to see how we used to work, and that our way of doing handover had become so normalised. The difference [following the implementation of the new handover practice] was enormous. I experienced the multidisciplinary feedback sessions as very pleasant, because you get a chance to talk with each other. Everyone looks at the footage from the perspective of their own profession, and when they talk about what they see, you learn from each other.'

Another recovery nurse commented:

> 'It [the video reflection method] is very appealing. You saw the previous situation and you saw how we changed things. Work becomes visible and it is not just theory telling you that if you do it differently it will be better. By visualising it [the work], we become a lot more involved and engaged. For me this [video feedback] has motivated me to continue with the new practice. I liked the multidisciplinary feedback sessions ... we were able to exchange experiences'.

Hospital 5: Improving paediatric cardiothoracic handover to the ICU

Hospital 5 is an academic paediatric hospital. Here, the participating research team focused on cardiothoracic surgery handovers at a paediatric ICU. This hospital performs more than 400 cardiothoracic surgeries each year.

During their focus group discussions, the anaesthesiologists and cardio surgeons characterised the post-surgery handovers at the paediatric ICU as uncertain and unsatisfactory. They felt that the intensive care nurses should be able to connect the patient in a more efficient way to the monitoring equipment. At the same time, the intensive care nurses talked about being aware of the anaesthesiologists and the cardio-surgeons at times being quite nervous and uncertain during these handovers. Especially the junior nurses were aware of this. This resulted in added stress for them and uncertainty about their own tasks and knowledge. To address these concerns, both the clinicians and the nurses agreed to video the post-cardiothoracic surgery handovers, to find out what could be done.

Upon viewing their own handover footage, the clinicians decided on a number of changes. First, the theatre nurses agreed that connecting the patient to the monitoring equipment could be done more efficiently. The preparation at the ICU while the patient was still under surgery was effective but not optimal. To improve this, the equipment should be set up at the ICU well before the patient's transfer.

Second, the infusion lines tended to be tangled up in and around the patient's crib, which made the transfer at the ICU difficult. Upon viewing the footage showing clinicians struggling with a mass of lines and cords that needed to be disconnected and reconnected, staff were reminded that a 'connector unit' had in fact been bought some time back and that this would allow simple and quick reconnection of a number of devices. When using this unit the various components of the monitoring equipment did not have to be transferred one by one, but could be connected all at once. This unit had never been implemented because this would have required making some minor technical changes to the equipment used. On viewing the footage, the clinicians realised the need for making these technical changes so that the connector unit could be used.

Third, the clinicians questioned whether the crib was really essential for transferring these newborns. They decided to use a normal bed, which would allow more working space.

A fourth intervention proposed by the nurses was that the verbal handover of the anaesthesiologists and the surgeons was often started while the nurses were still reconnecting the patient. They also felt that there were too many people around the bed, particularly when the patient still needed to be connected. A particular risk here was posed by visiting parents, usually brought along by the surgeons. This meant that the nurses were unable to pay full attention to the parents, or to the handover, resulting in problems. When viewing the footage, the medical clinicians realised that the nurses were unable to hear the verbal handover, sometimes because the nurses were busy reconnecting the patient and were therefore standing with their back towards the medical staff delivering the handover, and sometimes this was because of the talk going on between the doctors and the parents. The footage also revealed that several verbal handovers could be going on at the same time, making it easy for the recovery room clinicians to miss important information. The lack of clear signals marking the end of the handover further made people unsure about whether they had finished. The senior clinicians realised that this already complex situation was made still more complex by the verbal handover being exploited as a teaching opportunity for the junior doctors. Although this teaching aspect is essential in an academic hospital, it did risk producing a prolonged and even more disorganised verbal handover. Another problem that was revealed was that this extra educational information was rarely relevant for the nurses taking charge of the patient.

In response to these concerns, the team agreed to redesign their handovers as follows. The verbal handover was only allowed to commence after the patient was connected and the vital signs had become visible on the screen. The ICU nurse who was going to take care of the patient had to stop all his or her activities and pay full attention to what was being said. A second nurse was allowed to continue with connecting the patient, if that proved necessary. Both the ICU doctor and the clinical fellow were to be present when the verbal handover starts. It was also agreed that the surgeon should start with the verbal handover, to be followed by the anaesthesiologist's handover. Parents were not going to be allowed into the unit until after the conclusion of the handover.

Ten months after implementation of these new practices, Elizabeth and Bas came back to video a number of handovers. Upon viewing the footage, all participants agreed that they were very satisfied with the process. One nurse commented:

> 'You notice a considerable difference compared to 10 months ago. Now, I can say when I am ready and have time and are able to fully concentrate on what the anaesthesiologist has to say. Previously, you were busy and you might hear something [or not]'.

One of the anaesthesiologists commented:

> 'I now feel that it is quieter during the whole process. I think that it is therefore more efficient and fewer mistakes are being made. Not that we ever had major accidents, but there were some sloppy things. I am very pleased with this connector unit. It is much faster'.

Hospital 6: Improving adult cardiothoracic surgery handovers to the ICU

Hospital 6 is the largest teaching hospital in the Netherlands, with 1000 beds and more than 5300 employees. Here, the participating research team focused on adult cardiothoracic surgery handovers to ICU staff. Both the anaesthesiologists and the intensive care nurses acknowledged during the pre-video meetings that the post-cardiothoracic surgery handovers at the ICU were not optimal. On viewing their own handover footage, the anaesthesiologists realised that their current handover communication with the intensive care nurses was quite ineffective. Eye contact was almost completely non-existent and there was a lot of background noise. When ICU nurses reconnected the patient to the monitoring equipment during the handover, they had their back to the anaesthesiologist who was providing the information. It was unclear whether the intensive care nurses could hear what was being said and whether they understood the information. Questions were hardly ever asked.

Further, the narrative of the anaesthesiologist was often interrupted when there were problems with the transfer of the monitoring equipment. The intensive care nurses felt that there were too many people around the bed of the patient and that they were getting in the way. The footage graphically displayed how people continually had to walk around each other. Also, the professionals present during the verbal handover varied widely, and this created variation in the person to whom the anaesthesiologist would hand over: this could be the intensive care nurses, the intensivist or the clinical fellow. It was even possible that the anaesthesiologist provided the same information twice or even three times to different professionals in the order in which they arrived.

Viewing the video footage led to several changes. The clinicians decided they needed to clarify the timing, the place, the participants, the content and the ending of their handovers. First, the verbal handover should only start if and when the vital signs were available on the monitor screen. Second, verbal handover should take place at the desk placed at the 'foot end' of the bed and where the handover form could be filled out. Third, the anaesthesiologist, the clinical fellow and the intensive care nurse all had to be present when the verbal handover started. Fourth, there was to be eye contact to ensure the handover receiver could signal they understood what was being communicated. Fifth, the special form had to be filled in and used by the anaesthesiologist to transfer the information to the clinical fellow and the intensive care nurses. Last, each handover was to end with the question if all information was clear and whether there were any questions. If there were any details to be added or tasks to be carried out, they had to be noted on the form.

Concluding discussion

This overview of achievements across the six participating sites shows that each team was able to produce significant outcomes. It is important to emphasise that none of the teams needed to abort the project, whether because of lack of interest, divergent opinions, political sensitivity or insufficient evidence of practical benefit. The people interviewed expressed their interest in the approach and were explicit about the benefits it had produced for their sites.

In addition, Elizabeth and Bas' checking of the project's achievements several months later revealed that many of the changes originally produced from the study were still in place. Overall, as the comments cited earlier confirm, participants felt enabled by seeing their own ways of working from a new perspective, they felt strengthened as teams by being able to talk about issues that before had remained below the surface of their conscious awareness, they felt able to connect problems visible on screen to behaviours on the ward, and they were able to discuss issues in a positive and constructive way, avoiding blame and accusation for matters that appeared to be sub-ideal.

In effect, the footage connected the participants to a dimension of their own practices that they had learned to take for granted, regard as unchangeable, or at least experience as being beyond their conscious control. What the footage highlighted were the richness, the multidimensionality and the extraordinary potential for practice enhancement and practice intervention.

We suggest that making this richness, multidimensionality and enhancement potential tangible made possible four things. First, it made those participating aware that they were witnessing something quite extraordinary. What was visible on the screen was not just 'ordinary', everyday practice; here, practice revealed itself as an ongoing accomplishment of great complexity. This was evident from how *fascinated* the clinicians invariably were by watching themselves on screen.

Second, this realisation, in turn, led to participants being motivated and inspired to improve what they were witnessing. Admittedly, footage produced of the feedback sessions captured some people covering their faces in apparent or pretended despair at what they were seeing, but there were also many smiles, as well as much energy to propose solutions and make changes. The mere fact that the video footage never led to people throwing their hands in the air and saying, 'this is hopeless, there's no point doing anything about this', is proof that video footage confirmed for people the value of their own accomplishments, strengthening their commitment to enhancing an already robust practice.

Third, instead of focusing participants only on the enactment of a verbal handover and its compliance to a pre-established protocol, participants considered the context of the handover, the actions of those present, people's bodily and facial behaviours, the technologies and other resources needed for the patient transfer – all matters that are critical to enhanced communication. These behavioural and contextual aspects of handover are hard to capture when considering only the spoken dimensions of handover. The footage made these aspects visible, and thereby made them amenable to change.

Fourth, collective viewing of one's own practices and collectively discussing it are equally critical dimensions of video-reflexivity and exnovation. Viewing footage does not just involve the individual practitioner and produce personal realisations. On the contrary, seeing practice unfold on the screen highlights its habituated groundings and systemic (networked) dimensions.

Put differently, it shows people how what they do is carried as it were, and often motivated by what others do and by what has gone on before, rather than being driven by their own personal reasoning and conscious planning. The footage shows people that they are implicated in a play whose lines they know but are at pains to articulate when asked to do so. In that sense, they are enmeshed in a social dramaturgy (Burke, 1969) whose logic exceeds people's personal intentions and goals. Here, individuals' intentions and realisations matter less than collectives' determinations and agreements. This is because viewing their own footage and discussing practice with each other in this register strengthens practitioners' collective ability to intervene in their own practices. These kinds of discussions strengthen what Weick might call collective mindfulness (Weick, 2004, or what we have referred to using the term 'weave of shared commitments'.

For Weick, collective mindfulness manifests as the preoccupation with potential failure, the reluctance to simplify interpretations, sensitivity to unfolding processes, cultivation of resilience and willingness to organise around expertise (Weick, 2004: 195–6). Few proposals are available however for how to generate collective mindfulness in clinical teams. Discussions that promote collective mindfulness often remain silent on how to instil it in people, suggesting it may be a personality trait or a personal predisposition rather than something that can be learned.

What video-reflexivity shows, and this is particularly evident from the reactions and responses from the participants cited in this chapter, is that watching and discussing footage of people's own work heightens their sense of having things in common, it strengthens their feeling of being part of a weave of pre-existing commitments, and it brings to the fore the importance of their place in practice as a social-organisational dynamic. This, we suggest, is the basis of mindfulness.

The significance of mindfulness is that it is a dynamic, contentless resource or capacity. It can turn its strengths to anything that confronts and challenges the team. This is a critical point because it is mindfulness, and not the individual solutions listed above, that are of importance. Ultimately, the particular solutions devised in response to viewing video footage are never going to be self-sufficient and will not last forever. They need to be scrutinised on an ongoing basis to test and improve their effectiveness given the constant changes in patients, staffing, spaces and technologies. Therefore, it is not the solutions themselves but, rather, mindfulness that matters. People's capacity to scrutinise practice as it unfolds and question aspects of practice with colleagues is the most prominent and valuable contribution of video reflexivity, and the most important dimension of 'teamness'. This capacity harbours the most lasting benefit for clinicians, for their patients and for clinical practice improvement generally.

8

Designing an ambulance paramedic to emergency triage staff handover protocol for New South Wales, Australia

Co-authored with Chris Ball

Introduction

Effective handover between ambulance paramedics and emergency department (ED) personnel is critical to ensuring all information pertaining to the patient's care is appropriately transferred (Thakore and Morrison, 2001). Handover works when the expectations of ambulance staff and ED clinicians are aligned, and when there is agreement about what information needs to be handed over (London Ambulance Service, 2008). One way of aligning professionals' information expectations is through standardising their handover process. With a standardised handover, ambulance staff can prepare for what to say when handing over, and clinicians will be familiar with the general outline of what they will hear and know what to ask for in addition in specific circumstances.

Clinical handover was only recently put on the health reform agenda by health policymakers interested in patient safety (Jorm *et al.*, 2009). This was in response to *in situ* research (Evans *et al.*, 2010) and meta-analyses of root cause analysis investigations of incidents (Rabøl *et al.*, 2011) revealing that ineffective clinical handover in many health services acted as a cause of serious incidents. As is common across health care, these findings and analyses were seen as pointing to a need for across-the-board implementation of a standardised handover protocol.

Around the same time, Haig and colleagues published their seminal paper advocating the SBAR handover protocol. SBAR is an acronym that stands for 'Situation, Background, Assessment, Recommendations' (Haig *et al.*, 2006). SBAR was found to be effective in defence contexts, and Haig and colleagues argued it would equally suit clinicians. The simplicity of the protocol and the abstract nature of its components stood in its favour, and it certainly provides a simple solution to the problem of getting clinicians to standardise their handovers in a way that was uniform and clear. Since then, SBAR has become the handover protocol of choice among policymakers and across health care services (Australian Commission on Safety and Quality in Health Care, 2009; New South Wales Health, 2009).[18]

SBAR undoubtedly provides much needed support for nurses informing doctors, or for junior medical staff informing senior medical staff. However, its format is not necessarily one that suits all clinical scenarios and handover events. To some extent, this point was acknowledged by policy agencies in Australia allowing opportunities for clinicians to adapt SBAR to their particular needs. They were allowed to do so on the principle that their unique locales, skills and needs might require a slightly different approach to handover delivery. Allowing front-line professionals to adapt standards and guidelines to suit their specific purposes has been labelled 'flexible standardization' (Timmermans and Berg, 2003). The term flexible standardisation, rather than referring to the collaborative construction of *standards*, is more productively interpreted to refer to the collaborative construction of *systems* of practice. Here, 'systems' encompass process designs, protocols and checklists, as well as practices that mobilise and thereby *realise* those resources.

For that reason, we regard flexible standardisation to mean 'giving frontline staff a say in systems development', and it would be more appropriate as 'flexible systematisation'. Marking a critical development in policy thinking, flexible standardisation as a concept has now gained considerable traction in local health policy reform discourse (Australian Commission on Safety and Quality in Health Care, 2009) and in practice improvement training discourse (Iedema *et al.*, 2009d).

Given its general remit and hence its wide applicability, SBAR might at first glance be appropriate not just for in-hospital handovers but also for ambulance-to-hospital transfers. SBAR's suitability to the ambulance–emergency interface

---

18 Also see www.institute.nhs.uk/safer_care/safer_care/sbar_resources.html

is not self-evident, however. One problem is that SBAR requires the paramedic handing over to recommend a course of action to the person receiving the handover. In the context of ambulance paramedic–emergency department staff dynamics, such requirements may come up against emergency staff expectations that they deduce their own clinical recommendations. Emergency clinicians will want information about the injury and about what the paramedic did by way of treatment, but hospital staff generally want to make their own decisions about continued treatment. Moreover, ambulance patients may require a fast handover because of the seriousness of their injury. In that case, it will be critical to deal with the nature of the injury and the vital signs earlier rather than later. This also draws attention to the fact that information pertaining to ambulance patients generally needs to be pithy, hierarchised and targeted.

Be that as it may, if there is no agreement among paramedics and emergency staff about what information components are to be handed over, their handovers will remain unpredictable, and the potential for error will remain high. To obtain such an agreement, it is critical to involve all relevant stakeholders and obtain their opinions about these and related matters. Such deliberations can help map out the opportunities and constraints inherent in geo-demographic locales, organisational resources and departmental spaces. These opportunities and constraints will play a critical determining role in the systematisation of the handover process. As we have argued in previous chapters, shared deliberation of these issues among the actors and stakeholders involved will enable them to consider the strengths, shortcomings and improvement possibilities of existing practice.

It was on this basis that a project was initiated to systematise the ambulance-emergency handover process in New South Wales, Australia. Clinicians' involvement in the project was secured by presenting it to them as a 'video-reflexive ethnographic' study whose success and outcomes were contingent on their participation. As has been made clear in previous chapters, video-reflexive ethnography involves clinicians observing footage of themselves at work; openly discussing the strengths and shortcomings in what they do, and together redesigning what they do and say into a systematised process. This method ensures that clinicians gain an opportunity to analyse their own practices, share their sense of accomplishment about being able to carry off complex kinds of work in challenging circumstances, align their understandings about current problems and challenges, and, if needed, collectively design alternative ways of working.

In what follows, we describe this project and its achievements in detail (Iedema *et al.*, 2012b). We first provide some background to the project, and then detail its findings and achievements.

Background
. . . .

In 2010, the New South Wales Health Ministerial Taskforce for Emergency Care made available funding for a project that sought to standardise the handover process between ambulance paramedics and emergency clinicians.[19] The 'NSW Ambulance-to-ED Handover Project' described in this chapter was established to develop, implement and evaluate a handover protocol ensuring the smooth transfer of pre-hospital care into the acute setting. The project was considered important because reports had revealed there was persistent uncertainty and disagreement at the ambulance–emergency interface about what issues were to be handed over, by whom and to whom the information was to be handed over, what role the information should play in the care subsequently provided by emergency staff, and how emergency staff were to understand the limitations and constraints bearing on paramedics due to having access only to a small space in the ambulance, ruling out more sophisticated and technologically advanced kinds of treatment.

While there are trauma protocols available to guide ambulance handovers, such as MIST (Mechanism of injury, Injury, [vital] Signs, Treatment given) and AMPLE (Allergies, Medications, Past illnesses, Last meal, Events), these protocols do not accommodate all handover scenarios with which ambulance paramedics may be confronted. That leaves a good proportion of handovers (those that do not involve trauma patients) unaccounted for, leaving both paramedics and emergency staff guessing what kinds of issues should be conveyed, in what order and at what level of detail. Focus groups with ambulance and emergency personnel further revealed that SBAR was not deemed ideal for the ambulance– emergency interface. Comments referred to a lack of specificity, an order of items that does not reflect the frequent urgency of ambulance transfers, and undue emphasis on paramedic recommendations in a context where emergency clinicians are focused on developing hospital-specific clinical management plans.

The project described in this chapter sought to alleviate the existing handover uncertainties by enabling practitioners to design a protocol that applies to all ambulance–emergency handovers, trauma as well as non-trauma. The project was structured as a before-and-after intervention. Overall, it had the following five objectives.

---

19 Here we acknowledge Barbara Daly's and Sarah Hoy's roles in articulating the project's aims and goals.

1. To engage ambulance and ED clinicians in assessment of and reflection on real-time visual data;
2. To design an ambulance–ED handover standard / protocol that aligns with the NSW Health Safe Clinical Handover Standard Key Principles (New South Wales Health, 2009);
3. To integrate this ambulance–ED handover standard / protocol into practice;
4. To evaluate how clinicians' use of the designed standard / protocol adheres to the NSW Health Safe Clinical Handover Standard Key Principles;
5. To evaluate the practical impact of the designed standard / protocol on clinical safety.

Objective 1 makes clear that this project was designed as a form of 'participative enquiry' (Reason and Bradbury, 2008). We advocated for this approach knowing that clinicians want to understand the provenance of changes that are introduced to their ways of working. Clinicians also need to see a reason for introducing the changes into practice, and they need to know there is shared agreement about and enthusiasm for putting them into practice. For this to happen, clinicians need to be involved in the design of local solutions and service delivery changes. Without their involvement, none of these conditions obtain. Their involvement ensured the handover protocol was designed in a 'bottom-up' way, rendering structure sensitive to the needs and concerns of front-line paramedics and clinicians.

In adopting this approach, the project put into practice the HELiCS approach developed for the Australian Commission on Safety and Quality in Health Care National Clinical Handover Project (Iedema et al., 2009e; Iedema et al., 2009d). As flagged in the previous chapter, HELiCS sets out a front-line staff training programme that includes an elaborate rationale and procedure for bottom-up design, accompanied by video-based training resources (Iedema et al., 2009c; Iedema and Merrick, 2008), online materials (see www.safetyandquality.gov.au/) and research publications (Iedema and Merrick, 2012; Iedema et al., 2012b; Iedema et al., 2009e; Iedema et al., 2009d). Following HELiCS, the defining components of the project approach were defined as listed in Box 8.1.

In practice, the application of this approach meant that paramedics and emergency staff were consulted about what they regarded to be the advantages and disadvantages of established ways of working, and about the kinds of changes they would like to see introduced. Following on from these discussions, and after obtaining ethics approval from all organisations involved and consent from all paramedics and emergency staff participating in the project, 73 handovers were filmed, and video-reflexive sessions were conducted where selections of the resulting footage were shown to front-line staff. We also analysed the handovers in terms of duration, amount of repeated information, numbers and kinds of questions and eye contact.

Box 8.1 Main components of the ambulance–emergency handover protocol development approach

1. **Participation**: Ambulance and ED staff will be involved through interviews and focus groups in outlining their concerns about existing handover practice and help define the *principal touch points*.[20]
2. **Observation**: Existing handover practice will be observed by a researcher to locate the principal touch points in real-time practice in preparation for filming.
3. **Filming**: Real-time handover will be captured on film as a way of making the principal touch points visible.
4. **Reflexive sessions**: Ambulance and ED staff will be involved in mixed focus groups to confront real-time practice, generate learning and derive insight into how to redesign handover into a handover standard compatible with NSW health policy.
5. **Implementation**: Ambulance and ED staff will be involved in, first, simulated trials of the new handover standard and, second, real-time roll-out.
6. **Ongoing self-evaluation**: Ambulance and ED staff will be engaged in ongoing self-evaluation.[21]
7. **Dissemination and training**: Dissemination of the process leading to the production of the handover standard and the handover standard itself will occur by deploying video resources for general training and by involving front-line staff in training sessions at other hospital sites.

The feedback sessions were structured to elicit comments in response to both the footage and the analytical findings. The process was to generate consensus among paramedics and emergency staff about the ideal format for a handover protocol. The next section of this chapter explains how such consensus was achieved.

---

20 A 'touch point' is a facet of practice that study participants and researchers identify as problematic and in need of attention and redesign (Bate and Robert, 2007).
21 For example, through engaging junior staff in observational measurements for their clinical assessments, educationally supervised by their university or training agency.

Handover analysis and protocol elicitation

Pre-video focus groups

Pre-video focus groups were held to allow staff an open forum to talk about the problems that they recognised in their current handover practice. A total of 10 pre-video focus groups were held, each lasting between 1 and 1½ hours. Three were held at hospital site 1 with ED clinicians, three at hospital site 2 with ED clinicians, and four with paramedics from the Ambulance Service of New South Wales. These focus groups allowed staff an open forum to express their thoughts on handover and the detailed processes that are involved.

The pre-video focus groups served to highlight a number of key issues, with paramedics and ED clinicians raising slightly different points and concerns. ED clinicians identified the following points.

- The accuracy of information handed over varies because of the variety of patient presentations and approaches taken by paramedics.
- Triage category 1 and 2 patients deserve a period of 'hands off' (before initiating treatment) because all team members need to pay attention to the ambulance paramedic's handover.
- Clinical assessment at triage by nursing staff needs to be possible because it is critical to patient safety.
- Handover should contain a core of consistent information; however, the depth of information should be allowed to vary between handover at triage and handover at the bedside, with the latter involving a more comprehensive assessment and extended communication of the patient's history and potential trajectory.

The paramedics identified the following challenges.

- Triage processes need to be standardised because:
  - At times handovers need to be repeated to different staff.
  - Different ED clinicians may request different information.
  - Resuscitation handovers are made difficult by responsible ED staff not always being easily identifiable.
  - Hospitals may have different processes relating to incoming critical patients or 'code 3s', case sheets and hospital codes.
- Relationships and communication with ED clinicians were commented on as potentially being hampered because of their:

▶ Inadequate attention to and respect for paramedic staff communicating handovers.

▶ Limited appreciation of the space, time and resource constraints affecting the clinical decisions and practices of ambulance paramedics.

These points cover both substantive concerns (what is said/heard), and political-interpersonal ones (how are things said/heard). Both the substantive and the political-interpersonal concerns needed to be addressed and resolved. Therefore, the deliberation process was not just about the development of a handover protocol but also about the reinvention of a relationship such that paramedics and emergency clinicians could enact mutual respect and professional confidence. We considered addressing both the substantive and the political-interpersonal dimensions of the paramedic–emergency relationship to be critical to achieving and maintaining safe handover practice.

Observation and filming of practice

Observation of practice involved the researcher (Chris Ball) first observing *in situ* care practices and behaviours. When it was clear which aspects of practice deserved attention, when they should be filmed, who was comfortable with being filmed and how the filming could be done, real-time filming of handover communication was initiated. The filming focused on the local complexities and processes of practice that were identified during the focus groups, and ones that became evident during the researcher observation process.

The researcher spent a total of 4 weeks observing ambulance handovers in the ED. Observations commenced at hospital site 1, where the researcher spent 2 weeks. In total, 90 clinicians and paramedics consented to participate in the study. Besides observing practice, the researcher filmed 33 handovers during this period. At hospital site 2, 79 clinicians and paramedics consented to participate in the study. The researcher spent 2 weeks observing practice, and during that period filmed a further 40 handovers.

Reflexive feedback

The reflexive feedback meetings gave paramedics and ED clinicians the opportunity to see and comment on their own practices. ED clinicians identified the following issues from watching the footage.

● There were high levels of ambient noise interfering with the triage process.

● When several ambulance patients are waiting to be triaged, emergency clinicians may need to engage in a pre-triage process to identify and start treating high-urgency cases further down in the ambulance cue.

- Triage handovers may require less detailed information than do bedside handovers.
- Maintaining concentration of all present for the entirety of the paramedic handover is sometimes difficult.
- Although they *thought* they could multitask during handover, the footage revealed for them that this may not actually be possible, effective or safe.

For their part, the paramedics identified the following issues from watching the footage.

- There were high levels of ambient noise interfering with the triage process.
- Differences in handover procedure can lead to problems:
  - ❯ Failing to document information appropriately and effectively can be risky:
    — paramedic case sheets are not always tailored to enable paramedics to respond to in-hospital information demands;
    — sometimes paramedics do handover without reference to case sheets;
    — paramedics sometimes write information on their gloves to prevent loss of information.
  - ❯ Structuring of handover information is important:
    — the triage nurse has a limited time span and paramedics need to deliver all the key information clearly and at the start of their handover;
    — trauma teams expect a rapid and well-structured handover; if this is not forthcoming, clinicians may stop paying attention to the handover;
    — when clinicians ask questions, they may throw the paramedic delivering the handover off track, causing them to forget what has already been handed over.

Important by way of initial conclusion was that both professional groups acknowledged that their handover practice needed to be better structured, given more clarity, conducted in a quieter environment, and invested with greater interpersonal attention and respect (e.g. through eye contact). Both groups also raised other issues that did not appear to rate for the other group (e.g. 'paying attention to the whole handover'), and these issues would require careful mediation to come to a productive resolution.

Formal analysis of pre-intervention handover communication

The total of 73 pre-intervention handovers were formally analysed. The focus was to uncover existing trends in current patient handover practice. This analysis included examining the individual clinical information components that made up a whole handover, the non-verbal communication patterns (eye contact, body movements) and handover duration during triage and in the resuscitation bay, in acute, sub-acute and in the trolley-waiting bay. The data was then correlated relative to paramedic levels of expertise and the severity of the patients involved. The resulting data was also related back to the views expressed during the initial focus groups.

The analytical procedure was as follows. The video data was first broken down to reveal the clinical information components contained in the handover. These components included: patient identification, chief complaint, information relating to the complaint, vital signs, treatment, allergies, medications, medical history, social history and other information (including information provided by the patient, family or carer). Videoed handovers were analysed for the order in which these components were mentioned, and for their presence or absence. A critical finding here was that there appeared to be a 'tacit sequence' in the way paramedics presented their information; that is, an order governing the components that were handed over in many paramedics' handovers, despite the handovers being otherwise quite ad hoc and even at times totally disorganised.

This 'tacit sequence' became apparent as follows. In all the handovers (100%) paramedics identified the patient first; 70% then continued onto the chief complaint; 31% then expressed information that related to the chief complaint and 37% of paramedics then handed over the patients' vital signs. Other information components following on from this initial sequence (such as treatment given, allergies, current medications) were not handed over in any identifiable order. The basic, tacit structure found in existing handovers then, was 'IMI': Identification, Mechanism of injury or Medical complaint, Injury or Information pertaining to the complaint. Note that this means that the 'IMI' format was tacitly deployed in existing practice for both trauma and non-trauma handovers. The remaining information components (e.g. vital signs, treatment given, allergies) were mentioned in an unpredictable order, and frequently were not mentioned at all.

Other findings included the following. First, triage clinicians asked questions either during or at the end in more than half of all handovers. This would not be a problem were it not that just under half of those questions were for information that had already been provided by the paramedic during the handover. This finding pointed to difficulties with ED clinicians comprehending and/or hearing paramedic information.

Second, it was evident that during handover, paramedics repeated information in a third of all handovers. A quarter of these repeats occurred after being asked a question by the clinician (requesting information to be repeated). Of all the questions asked by clinicians during handover, a quarter of their questions occurred after a paramedic had already repeated information. This revealed a potential waste of both paramedics' and ED clinicians' time and resources.

Third, handover length was found to vary greatly. The shortest handover recorded was 26 seconds and the longest was 248 seconds. Both higher acuity of the patient and juniority of the paramedic handing over were found to contribute to longer handover duration.

Fourth, eye contact was discovered to be a key factor affecting handover length. Interestingly, and reminiscent of a related finding of the Utrecht study presented in Chapter 7, the length of time was found to decrease depending on the level of eye contact engaged in during the handover process. If there was eye contact for greater than 30% of the total handover, this eye contact was found to co-occur with a lower average handover length of 85 seconds (Iedema *et al.*, 2012b).

Handover protocol development

Reflexive focus groups were convened so that the researchers could present to ambulance paramedics and ED clinicians both the video footage of existing practice and the initial analytical findings. This feedback meeting sought to achieve another critical outcome: staff reflexivity. Reflexivity involved staff in commenting on and exploring the change potential of their own handover practice. Footage of real-time handovers was edited for presentation at these reflexive feedback meetings in compliance with institutional ethics requirements. The edited footage included five exemplars of handover practice, with each clip lasting less than 3 minutes.

This reflexive methodology proved to be a powerful means for staff to see the need for a change in handover practice, and to identify ways of achieving change. All health professionals involved in the project were invited to comment on their current practice and explore possibilities for improvement. This meant that the discussion was less about espoused positions and accepted knowledge than about what was visible in, evident from and made possible by the real-time video footage. These discussions enabled paramedics and ED clinicians to agree that the tentative structure already evident in how they currently delivered their handovers (and demonstrated by the formal analysis of the first batch of videoed handovers) should be emphasised; that specific components should be made more salient and others added; that some space should be given to questions and comments in order to make the handover more dialogic, and that specific body comportments should be prescribed to ensure they raise the effectiveness of the communication process.

As it seemed so well embedded in existing practice, the tacit 'IMI' structure was assumed as needing to be the basis of the new handover protocol. This was because we did not want to subvert or change too radically existing aspects of practice that worked for paramedics. Doing so might have meant the proposed change would have fallen on fallow ground, and been ignored. Another factor in favour of 'IMI' was its already existing application to both trauma and non-trauma cases. Thirdly, 'IMI' is reminiscent of 'MIST', a well-known ambulance handover protocol, albeit reserved to date for trauma patients.

Extending out from this tacit structure, the handover protocol was complemented with information components that paramedics and ED clinicians saw as critical to ambulance handover. These components were derived through analysis of what was most often repeated during handovers, and of what was most frequently asked, albeit in unpredictable ways. Thus, for example, critical was 'treatment given (by the paramedic)', 'medications that the patient was already taking', 'background of the patient', and 'allergies'. Extended deliberation among the researchers produced no viable solution other than complicated acronyms that looked like alphabet soups. Then, Chris Ball had the good fortune to meet Jacinta Young, an intensive care paramedic from Urunga, northern New South Wales. Jacinta mentioned that she had done a project on ambulance–emergency handover and that she had struggled to develop a handover mnemonic. She told Chris that she had had a flash of insight early one morning: IMISTAMBO. Miraculously, IMIST-AMBO matched our analyses of the video footage and resonated with our syntheses of paramedics' and clinicians' comments made during the reflexive meetings.

Where Jacinta's acronym was based on an early morning hunch, we were able to furnish research evidence for its suitability and applicability. We were further able to argue that IMIST-AMBO (we explain the significance of the hyphen below) can cater for the handover of trauma and of general patients. The trauma/non-trauma IMIST-AMBO mnemonic was subsequently defined as follows: I, Identification; M, Mechanism/Medical complaint; I, Injuries/Information relating to the complaint; S, Signs; T, Treatment and Trends; A, Allergies; M, Medication; B, Background history; and O, Other information.

The formulation of IMIST-AMBO accomplished agreement on the substantive structure of the paramedic–ED clinician handover. Four further issues were identified during the focus groups and feedback meetings as critical to how and where IMIST-AMBO is delivered.

1. The hyphen between IMIST and AMBO indicates a moment of pause (1–2 seconds recommended) where the paramedic can now expect questions and comments from the triage clinician.
2. The handover is to be an interruption-free zone.
3. 'Hands off, Eyes on': 20 seconds are to be reserved for the paramedic to convey IMIST-AMBO. During this 20-second period, ED clinicians are not to handle the patient or equipment, and are to grant the paramedic a modicum of eye contact to ensure there is 'shared attention'.
4. ED staff role identification: the trauma team leader needs to ensure they can be easily identified for paramedic handover – for example, medical and nursing team leaders are to wear blue gowns.

The IMIST-AMBO protocol was ratified by the Ambulance-to-ED Clinical Handover Expert Reference Group overseeing the project, and this meant we could move on to trialling, training and evaluating the protocol.

Protocol trial and training

The new protocol was then trialled at both hospital sites. Because of the large number of paramedics that may be present at each ED, the researcher met with members from education and area management from the Ambulance NSW. It was agreed that a 'cluster training' approach would be most effective. This approach involved training paramedics and ED staff at work and on the spot, filming their new handover practice, and giving 'hot feedback' about their new handover practice. This 'hot feedback' involved staff being given an impression about how they performed the new protocol immediately after having been instructed in its format and then enacting it as part of their patient handover. To further assist in generating compliance with and awareness of the protocol, 10 large IMIST-AMBO signs and 500 pocket-sized and plastic-coated IMIST-AMBO cards were prepared for distribution.

At hospital site 1, 60 clinicians and 118 paramedics were trained in the new protocol. This targeted training and feedback took place over 3 weeks. The same process unfolded at hospital site 2 and lasted 2 weeks. During this period, 48 clinicians and 102 paramedics were trained at site 2, or a total of 150 staff. A further 45 paramedic educators were also trained in the protocol. The grand total of staff trained across both sites was 373 over a total of 5 weeks (373 constitutes over 10% of the total number of paramedics currently employed in New South Wales).

More specifically, the training and feedback processes involved the following. At hospital site 1, the researcher and a clinical training officer attended the ED each day for the first week of protocol implementation. Both engaged paramedics in on-site training during times of bed-block when paramedics were forced to wait. At site 2, an area liaison officer assisted in recruiting paramedics for training. Another training opportunity offered itself when paramedics waited to be assigned to a new job. Training staff during periods of bed-block and while waiting for task assignment meant that each training session was limited to around 5 minutes. To increase awareness of the protocol, the researcher also gave a lecture to around 45 educators from around the state. This lecture sparked a large amount of discussion on the topic and several requests for information about the protocol. For their part, the researcher gave medical and nursing ED clinicians on-the-spot training during in-service times, bedside teaching sessions and medical teaching sessions.

Evaluating the new protocol

Evaluation of the protocol was achieved by utilising video-ethnographic methods in combination with a five-question survey. With regard to the former, and upon completion of the protocol training and *in situ* feedback, paramedics were given an average of a 1-week period before they were videoed as part of the evaluation process. During this period, 31 handovers were videoed at hospital site 1 and 33 at hospital site 2, yielding a total of 64 videoed handovers. Further, consenting of participants was also required because of some staff not having been present when the researcher originally obtained the consent of clinicians to do the videoing. The total number of participants in the study who had given consent was 67 ED clinicians and 224 paramedics. The impact of the video feedback, the training and the *in situ* feedback were assessed by analysing the video footage of the post-intervention handovers, and by comparing analytical findings to those produced from the pre-intervention video footage analysis.

Order and frequency

An analysis was done of the post-intervention handovers with regard to what was handed over and in what order (Iedema *et al.*, 2012b). This analysis shows that I[dentification of the patient] was spoken about first in all handovers analysed (pre-intervention: also 100%); M[edical complaint] or M[echanism] were presented second in 97% of all handovers (pre-intervention: 63%). Injury/

Information about complaint was mentioned third in 98% of handovers (pre-intervention: 55%), and vital signs was mentioned in fourth position in 65% of all post-intervention handovers (pre-intervention: 36%). The remaining elements of the handover protocol were still delivered with quite some unpredictability, but all information components saw an increase in the number of times they were mentioned.

Handover duration

Another critical point is that this increase in the amount of information that is handed over did not come at the cost of increasing the length of time required to deliver the handover. The length of pre-intervention handovers was, on average, 96 seconds. Post intervention decreased to an average length of 83 seconds. This has resulted in a saving of 13 seconds and a decrease in handover length by 13.5%. This decrease in time is significant when compared with the amount of admissions to hospital by ambulance each day. Site 2 has had up to 80 ambulances arrive in one 24-hour period. With a saving of 13 seconds, this would create a spare 17 minutes for ED clinicians for other tasks.

Questions asked after handover

Questions were asked in 56% of pre-intervention handovers, and in 41% of post-intervention handovers. Of the pre-intervention questions, 46% requested information that had already been handed over. Post-intervention, only 15% of questions asked requested information that had already been given. These changes can be interpreted as introduction of the protocol not only decreased the need to ask questions but also increased ED clinicians' retention and comprehension of information.

This marked increase in comprehension could be due to a multitude of factors addressed by means of the protocol. A critical role here may be played by the increased predictability of the kind and placing of the information given, the creation of a specific point at which ED clinicians can now ask questions (during the 2-second break between IMIST and AMBO), and the improvement in the amount of eye contact between the handing-over paramedic and the clinician receiving the information (as explicitly prescribed by the protocol). There was also a marked decrease with regard to information being repeated by paramedics during handover after a question had been asked: paramedics repeated information pre intervention 22% of the time, compared with only 8% post intervention. This drop may be due to the paramedics now having a set order to follow for their handover with set times and places for ED clinician questions (minimising confusion caused by being asked questions at unexpected moments). Post intervention, and upon being asked questions, paramedics were more easily able to revert back to their original place in the handover protocol.

The survey questionnaire that was distributed to emergency clinicians was printed on e-tablets that fed data directly into an e-database daily. The survey had five questions, eliciting emergency clinicians' views on whether and how paramedic handovers had improved. ED clinicians were asked to fill out the survey after receiving a handover both before and after the study intervention. The tablets contained five questions, each allowing for four answers: (1) strongly agree, (2) agree, (3) disagree and (4) strongly disagree.

The tablets were supposed to perform daily downloads of response data. However, often this feature was not working and required manual downloads by staff at the hospital. Because of workload pressures, these manual downloads were not always done. The tablets also required daily recharging. This meant that tablets often went for days without being recharged, as there was not always someone able to perform this task. Because of these factors, the data yield was more limited than planned during some periods of the study.

These limitations notwithstanding, 53% of clinicians strongly agreed before the intervention that the paramedic handover contained sufficient information. Post intervention, this figure went up to 63%. On the question as to whether the information was structured in the correct order of importance, pre-intervention confirmative answers were 45% and post-intervention answers were 55%. The remaining responses showed less convincing improvements. This was possibly because emergency clinicians were giving feedback on all of the paramedics they encountered, and not merely the ones trained as part of the present project. Given 10% of the paramedics were trained, clinicians' responses pertained to handovers given by paramedics aware of the protocol and ones who had not yet had the opportunity to familiarise themselves with the protocol. Considered overall, clinicians' feedback was mildly positive, pointing to the need for broader deployment of the protocol and more systematic evaluation.

Conclusion

This project is an example of protocol development that draws on the insights of front-line staff, on the skills and habits embedded in their daily practice, and on their energy and commitment to improving their own practices. In deploying this project and its unique approach, the researchers lent credibility to anthropologists' dictum that actors often have good reasons for acting as they do (Garfinkel, 1967), and that changing the bases of action must start with them, their habits and their reasoning. While much 'culture research' sets store by casting actors in terms of fixed attitudes, norms and beliefs, the approach deployed here made evident that actors were more than capable of evaluating their own practices, intervening in them, and changing their habits and relationships in the interest of values and norms they all hold dear.

Claims about cultural inertia and the like may therefore be no more than a logical restriction flowing forth from the constraints inherent in culture research itself. Such constraints are readily apparent in the survey questionnaire method, and in the way it fixes actors' stances and intentionality. The account given here reveals that, persistent problems notwithstanding, professionals are capable of reinventing their own ways of working once made aware of their taken-as-given habits and their potential for change. Given the opportunity, they will show themselves capable of reflexivity and process redesign.

Another point that bears repeating is that the focus of the present project – a new handover protocol – is not defining of what the project produced. Rather, what is defining of this research is that front-line professionals are enabled to 'see themselves from under a different aspect' (Iedema *et al.*, 2009e). This change in perspective is essential for learning and for a change in people's relationships and identity. Besides throwing light on how we do handover, this realisation that there are alternative perspectives on what we do and who we are is critical for expanding the activity space – the zone of practice – of practitioners. Learning, in this context, is transformational – not merely in a cognitive or personal sense, where I can now experience myself differently and more acutely, but also in a social-organisational sense, where we experience the quality and significance of our work relationships with greater acuity. This, we suggest, generates a meta-discourse – a shared way of talking *about* everyday practice. This meta-discourse is a critical resource as it enables practitioners to bond, not so much through discussing interpersonal issues, as through discussing work-related issues. We believe such meta-discourse is the condition of origin of what Weick calls 'collective mindfulness' (Weick, 2004). However, we acknowledge that mindfulness may encompass *affect* (a hard to articulate sense of significance and connection), over and beyond explicit discourse.

Mindfulness arises from professionals having faith in the strength of their relationships to such an extent that they feel 'carried' by those relationships. Such feeling of being 'carried' by others (and of being able to 'carry' others) arises when people close-by know what I may not know and I know I can call on them. This mutual feeling creates a zone of safe practice, a zone where my uncertainties and imperfect actions can be shared with and checked by others without incurring sanction and recrimination. Such a zone is also critical for senior experts who are able and willing not just to teach but also learn from their more junior staff.

In the next and final chapter of this book, we will bring these and related issues together in our overarching argument. We therefore have to shift gears again, but now from people's everyday experiences and *in situ* examples back towards generalisation and theory. We will pick up again some of the themes set out in the first four chapters in this book, but now informed by and enhanced with the achievements and learnings set out in this second part of the book.

9

Conclusion

Improving one's own practices and relationships 'from within'

Reprise: exnovation as innovation 'from within'

This book has been about exnovation using video-reflexive ethnography. Let us summarise what we have said about the point and focus of this approach.

- It acknowledges that front-line clinicians[22] embody resources and capacities (such as vigilance, resilience, adaptive action and reflexive practice) that are critical to health care quality and safety.
- It posits that people are likely, if shown visual or other evidence portraying their own *in situ* ways of acting, to appreciate anew the richness and complexity of their practices.
- It capitalises on this realisation to focus people on aspects of practice that they would otherwise regard as taken as given, and therefore as not in need of change or as unavailable for change (because taken as given).
- It harnesses the affective impact of visual footage to motivate people to collectively reshape practices and relationships in ways that intervene in not just knowing-that, but also knowing-how, including political, cultural and hierarchical conducts and routines.
- It enables people to identify opportunities for change that align with what they do, understand the rationales underpinning the proposed changes, and

---

22 We consider patients also play a critical role here. Because this book has not focused on co-design involving patients (Iedema *et al.*, 2010), but merely on practitioners, we will restrict our concluding comments to practitioners.

put these changes more quickly into practice than ones that are invented by 'experts elsewhere' and imposed from above.

- It balances out the conventional focus on ensuring front-line practitioners enact 'evidence-based practice' by crediting them with the capacity to co-produce 'practice-based evidence' (Horn and Gassaway, 2007).

- It expands the definition of 'practice-based evidence' (Horn and Gassaway, 2007) by framing 'practice-based evidence' as going beyond people collectively articulating their knowing-how for the purpose of generating new guidelines for others elsewhere, to people collectively building, updating and inventing new kinds of collective competence for and among *themselves*.

- It posits that this activity of scrutinising one's own practice and deriving new action principles for that practice engenders, nurtures and strengthens people's distributed intelligence.

- Distributed intelligence manifests in the form of not just *ad hoc* solutions produced through team resilience, but also as locally designed solutions through which practitioners rationalise and strengthen their own ways of working.

- Locally designed solutions, far from exacerbating specific sites' or practices' idiosyncrasies and risks, underwrite clinicians' and patients' own safety expectations, technical-clinical quality and safety standards, as well as the evolving demands of health reform (as the examples in this book have shown).

In this book, the focus has not been on how clinical activity falls short of idealised criteria, procedures and protocols. Instead, we have focused on uncovering and highlighting the richness of existing practice, and giving people confidence in recognising and mobilising the change potential of practice. We have been interested in the richness of existing practice and the already-present acumen that is embedded in and evident from *in situ* practice. That is, our focus has been on how front-line actors negotiate the complexity of *in situ* practice, on the often tacit resources they harness to do so, and on their capacity for confronting workplace complexity and for designing work processes in more considered ways.

This focus on the accomplishment and preservation of safety is of utmost importance. It deserves more attention in patient safety research than is the case to date, as much of this research targets incidents and errors.

The problem with existing approaches to incident classification and incident investigation: deficit thinking

Focusing on incidents and errors as the basis for improvement means adopting a deficit view on clinical practice. Those who espouse deficit thinking assume that concentrating exclusively on incidents and errors will yield fruitful solutions ensuring practice improvement. Deficit thinking suffers from major drawbacks (Dekker, 2005; Mesman, 2009). One is the idea that incidents can be reconstructed and that such reconstructions will reveal clear-cut 'root causes' (the 'hindsight problem'). Another is that such focus on incidents ignores the remainder of practice where several taken-as-given routines can be in operation that may well have contributed to the incident (we look for causes in carefully circumscribed places much as we 'look for our keys under the streetlight'). Yet another is that deficit thinking privileges not individuals' experiences, but a bureaucratically defined notion of 'incident'.

An important dimension of deficit thinking is that it emasculates itself before it has effect. Thus, incident classification and investigation are to avoid 'blaming individuals'. In adopting this 'detached' orientation, incident classification and incident investigation instigate radical segregations between what individuals do and experience *in situ* and what individuals need to talk about to understand and fix the problem. Put differently, by excising personal experience from incident classification and incident investigation, these initiatives divorce what happened from who did what – a move that disappoints and frustrates patients who are harmed no end (Iedema *et al.*, 2011, 2012). This separation gives rise to two serious problems: individuals are unable to discuss and understand their specific roles in what happened, and, as a consequence, individuals are unable to take action with respect to themselves and their actions in their attempt to obviate incidents. All they can do is subscribe to generalised aims and initiatives promising systems change.

This situation is problematic. What is needed instead is practitioners and patients being enabled to discuss incidents and errors within the context of their unique experiences (Dekker 2005, 2008, 2011). Articulating one's experiences is critical to being able to make sense of what happened, and establish common ground about what happened with others. If they do talk about their experiences, people may learn about aspects of what they do that are central to causing incidents, and others that are critical to avoiding incidents.

In engaging in such talk, they may develop a *meta*-discourse about the clinical work (Iedema *et al.*, 2009e). Such meta-discourse does not erase individuals' experiences, but foregrounds them and acknowledges them, weaving them into (and ensuring they are compatible with) team-based agreements governing the work.

> Such an approach would mean that incidents and errors are classified and investigated in ways that take account of the experiences of those involved in such problems, both clinicians and patients. These experiences need not be all negative, and they may harbour critical clues to how to avoid problems in the future.

Most of the time, practitioners keep work processes and tasks relatively safe. They do so by navigating through unpredictability, uncertainty and sometimes adversity. Their skills make up what Aristotle termed 'phronesis' (Flyvbjerg, 2001). As detailed in Chapter 2, phronesis is a learned and (over time) naturalised practical knowing-how-to-act. For experts, phronesis or knowing-how can become taken for granted, tacit, and thereby invisible (Dreyfus, 1979). Its taken-for-grantedness puts it beyond reach, and renders it inflexible. In these cases, phronesis risks becoming a private resource, potentially denying others benefit from it and a role in it.[23] Video, we have suggested, intervenes in this situation on two fronts.

First, viewing video footage shows practitioners how entangled they are as individuals in established ways of doing and saying. Viewing video footage of their own work reveals how their actions and decisions issue forth from a collective flow of activities – from *practice*. While people may focus on themselves and their actions in the footage, their attention will inevitably be on how they *interact* with others, how others interact with them, and what the dynamics are of that interaction. They apprehend themselves therefore not as monadic individuals acting out personal traits, but as socially enmeshed *interactants*. They see themselves as entangled in the complex dynamics of practice that more often than not supersede their own reasoning and conscious intentions.

This sense of *entanglement* comes about, on the one hand, by people becoming aware that responsibility for what occurs is inevitably dispersed across the group. Here, responsibility refers to 'an obligation to answer for what occurs'. The video footage shows them that what they do is not purely an effect of their personal making or their private intent, but also (and often overwhelmingly) an effect of how *practice works*. Answering for what occurs therefore would involve referring to 'how things are done around here', and saying, 'but this is how I am expected to act and behave'. On the other hand, this entanglement comes about through people gaining a sense of accountability. Accountability refers to 'the imperative to describe (offer an account about) what occurs'. Through viewing

---

23 Sloterdijk writes about the significance of actors in the modern world developing the capacity to participate in others' competence ('Teilhabe an Fremdcompetenz'; Sloterdijk, 2009: 594).

themselves in action, people become more able to offer an account about what happens.

To put this point slightly differently, upon viewing video footage of themselves at work, people's sense of being personally and causally implicated in ongoing actions tends to recede, while their ability and willingness to talk about their and others' actions tends to strengthen. The video-reflexivity meetings reported in previous chapters have offered ample examples of this. The sheer number of projects and positive outcomes presented confirm that viewing footage of *in situ* practice encourages social bonding (we are collectively responsible for what occurs here) as well as articulacy (we can find words to talk about what occurs here).

Second, viewing video footage of our own work brings the taken-for-granted dimensions of our expertise back into view. This enables practitioners to reappraise their expertise against contemporary knowledge, technologies and constraints. Such reappraisal enables everyone to talk about what is expertise and learn from it. Negotiating the substance and essence of expertise in this way establishes for all stakeholders a new platform of shared meaning and feeling that acts as a springboard into further learning. Framed thus, exnovation is making the phronesis of experts and the phronetic needs of novices visible, tangible and open to intervention, recreation and reinvention.

What is more, making practitioners' expertise (their phronesis) visible and tangible is important not only for raising their awareness of entanglement and enabling reappraisal of their own expertise. It is also important for showing that expertise that has become taken as given, or tacit, may lose its capacity to develop, as well as its capacity to usefully inform and interact with novices. Such expertise (particularly if it is wedded to organisational and professional authority and hierarchy) may have calcified into unquestioned, intractable habits. Writing early in the twentieth century, John Dewey maintained that we encounter the world in the first instance through our habits, not through conscious perceptions or explicit cognitions: 'Concrete habits do all the perceiving, recognizing, imagining, recalling, judging, conceiving and reasoning that is done' (Dewey, 1922: 130).

Encountering the world through habits means the following: we tend to judge people, initiate actions and negotiate events on the basis of taken-as-given notions, norms and activities. This way of being in the world may leave our habits themselves unquestioned, even in circumstances where it is they, rather than the obstacles we encounter in our path, that are the source of our trouble. Video viewing brings habits into view and makes them available for reconsideration.

Viewing video distances things and brings things closer

● ● ● ● ● ● ● ● ● ● ●

By viewing ourselves on video we make our habits visible and tangible. In doing so, we distance ourselves from unquestionably accepting our habits as an adequate basis for engaging in action and judging experience. The distancing at issue here is a process described by philosopher Peter Sloterdijk (2009) in terms of 'secession'. Secession refers to people's distancing from their social background, their social home base. He also uses the term 'recession' which refers to people distancing from their self- and identity-defining habits. For Sloterdijk, secession and recession are becoming defining capabilities for people in the twenty-first century. This is because the contemporary world is increasingly fast-changing and therefore unstable. Our habits are more rapidly 'out of date', and more rapidly in need of being reinvented. In essence, social-personal distancing enables us to reassess the 'fit' between our habits and the complexity of circumstances that we face. Through such distancing, the efficacy of our own ways of being and acting, and the complexities of everyday life, are opened up for interrogation and re-invention.

In proposing exnovation as a means to effect such distancing, we reconfirm the idea that practitioners themselves are not just a critical source of innovation but also an effective source of change. Practitioners do more than act out or 'make fit' established guidelines, and when they are obstructed in doing so, they will do more than show resilience to salvage the situation as best they can, or plan ahead to avoid similar problems. Seen from the perspective of exnovation, front-line staff are capable of *emergent, adaptive conduct that comes to inform future conduct*. This is conduct that may have no logical explanation and no rational link to what went before (Sloterdijk, 2009). It may transcend expectations, because it may go well beyond what was considered possible.[24] Think back to the neonatal intensive care nurses challenging the doctors about interrupting their workflow, the surgeons and anaesthesiologists agreeing to wait for the nurses to reconnect the patients and signal readiness for the handover, or the ambulance paramedics and emergency personnel agreeing on a behavioural regime of handover communication. These are examples of creative, norm-breaking inventions.

Video-reflexivity is therefore not merely a means to achieve innovation of practice. It constitutes a practice-improvement pedagogy for those at the sharp end of

---

24 The cover image on Sloterdijk's book, titled 'You have to change your life' (*Du mußt dein Leben ändern: Über Anthropotechnik*) represents an instance of how humans can exceed expectations – in this case, a single person holding up 10 others, forming an inverted human pyramid.

practice. Lillrank and Liukko's broom diagram (*see* Figure 2.1) showed that not just plans but also ad hoc decisions and dynamically changing decisions – and not just prefigured practices but also one-off actions – make up the profile of *in situ* activity. The implication of this last point is that frequently front-line staff make things up as they go, juggling mounting clinical tasks, technical and resource constraints, constant interruptions, piles of paperwork, and trading risks, competing demands, and compromises. Given they are embedded in practice in this multilayered way, practitioners are best placed to make sense of the constraints and the *possibilities* inherent in their own work. They need to be enabled to learn so they can take advantage of those possibilities and potentials.

Not surprisingly, when practitioners turn to watch their own ways of working, they are able to devise solutions that are not *exogenous* (external) but *endogenous* (germane) to who they are and to what they are already doing. This is where the distancing effect of video viewing splices into the contrary effect of bringing things closer: video viewing generates solutions that emerge from the existing practice potential. These solutions are not designed by experts elsewhere, imposed on events everywhere. Rather, they are incremental modifications that are sensitive to the constraints, problems and potentials embedded in prevailing activities, identities, resources and circumstances. Video footage re-portrays these activities, identities, resources and circumstances, and thereby alerts people to what is, and to what is possible and necessary.

Critical now is that we nurture professional practitioners who can become reflexive in this way and capitalise on what is possible. To do so, they must be open to what is possible and necessary: they must be capable of being affected by that which surrounds them and by those who work with them. For that reason, the pedagogies that we deploy in health for practice improvement must radically change. Instead of training clinicians in 'detached concern', we need to train them in becoming responsive beings – people attuned to those around them. As quoted at the beginning of Chapter 1:

> The education of the new professional will reverse the academic notion that we must suppress our emotions in order to become technicians . . . We will not teach future professionals emotional distancing as a strategy for personal survival. We will teach them instead how to stay close to emotions that can generate energy for institutional change, which might help everyone survive. (Palmer, 2007, cited in Berwick, 2009: w562)

Here an important distinction becomes apparent. Whereas traditional approaches to the professionalisation of clinicians centred on their distancing from the other (viz. 'detached concern'), exnovation requires the exact opposite: distancing from self. However, distancing from self is not about the annihilation of emotions, but about their recognition and harnessing to more intelligent futures.

Objections to and arguments for video-based practice improvement

There are detractors who regard video footage as incapable of adequately capturing the systemic problems facing health care. Their three main objections to using video for practice improvement were discussed in Chapter 4. With the benefit of the practical evidence presented in Chapters 5–8, let us briefly revisit these objections and strengthen our rebuttals.

The first was that video footage provides little more than a narrow perspective on practice. Here is a recent instance of such objection:

> Doctors only 'see' a fraction of the care they give . . . sometimes this is literally so but there is a broader system, *not so easily videotaped*, where doctors' action and inaction, particularly their disengagement from system improvement and management, results in patients suffering poor care and adverse events. (Jorm, 2012: 19; our italics)

This objection regards video as incapable of revealing anything other than strictly local activity. For that reason, and because it is impossible to film all aspects of practice, video footage is taken to be, as per definition, unrepresentative of practice. In Chapter 4, this objection was argued to be motivated by the naïve realist stance that in principle it *is* possible to see a 'view from nowhere' that can take in everything everywhere.

This naïve stance buttresses two related and deeply problematic ideas. One is that some approaches, such as large sample studies and controlled trials, are superior in their access to and representation of 'the real', because unfettered by the local, narrow and 'subjective' focus that defines, for example, video-ethnographic enquiry. It is further part of this belief that scientific representation, particularly numerical representation, is less constrained as a sign-based or 'semiotic' system than are other systems (language, or visuality). Scientific representations should therefore be seen, so this argument goes, as providing more accurate access to the totality of 'the real' than do other methods of representation.

As systems of representation, language, visuality and numbers clearly have different affordances; that is, they do different kinds of work. However, not one of these systems can lay claim to having a greater or better grip on 'the real'. The main difference in affordance among these systems of representation is not a supposed unequal capacity to make truth claims about 'the real'. On the contrary, their difference in affordance pertains to the varying degrees of generalisation and specification that they make possible. Numbers generalise, visuality specifies, and language can do both, depending on the uses to which it is put (Iedema *et al.*, 2003).

Our concern in this book (*see* Chapter 4 in particular) has been to point out that specification, achieved through visualising and narrating local events and unfoldings, is an increasingly critical resource and capability for understanding the fine-grained differentiations needing to be recognised when acting amidst complexity. Visualisation and narrative language therefore are increasingly important resources for acting amidst complexity.

The other problem produced by the 'view from nowhere' stance is the idea that we need to continue to produce more knowledge and evidence, that more knowledge and evidence will fill in gaps in what we know, and that more knowledge and evidence are needed before we can act or can decide how to act. This 'we must first fill the gaps in our knowledge' argument is responsible for fettering us to a Sisyphean task – a task that will never end. Such a task is impossible for two reasons. We will never be able to tell whether we are progressing, and we will never know enough to start the task. Put succinctly, we will never know everything there is to know. Even if we did come to know everything, it would rapidly go out of date, given the speeds at which life and knowing travel. For that reason, at a local level, actors are increasingly having to invent what they know together rather than pull knowledge off the shelf and apply and implement it. This is where 'the view from nowhere' (Nagel, 1989) runs up against 'the end of certainty' (Prigogine, 1996).

> [W]e believe that we are actually at the beginning of a new scientific era. We are observing the birth of a science that is no longer limited to idealised and simplified solutions but reflects the complexity of the real world, a science that views us and our creativity as part of a fundamental trend present at all levels of nature. (Prigogine, 1996: 7)

The second objection commonly raised against video was that the camera induces the 'Hawthorne effect'. Video is assumed to affect practitioners to the point where they will modify their practices in the knowledge they are being videoed. This objection was countered earlier in the book by saying, first, that practitioners' attempts at modifying their practice are invariably short-lived because people find it difficult to act in ways other than those to which they are habituated. The second point made was that the aim of video-reflexivity is precisely for people to learn to see themselves and others as outsiders might. If anything, and far from trying to downplay the significance of the Hawthorne effect, our stance involves capitalising on the self-consciousness that comes with the Hawthorne effect – also referred to as 'reflexivity'. Indeed, we advocate rendering the Hawthorne effect a *constant* in front-line service providers' thinking and behaviour.

For those who have used video footage for reflexive purposes, these objections founder not just because of the counterarguments that we just rearticulated. They also founder because of the enormous practical impact that video has on practice. The effect of video goes well beyond inciting protective behaviour aimed at making a good impression on the part of those claimed to be subject to the Hawthorne effect. Confirming earlier studies (Carroll *et al.*, 2008; Iedema *et al.*, 2009e; Neuwirth *et al.*, 2012), every project discussed in this book has shown that the effects on people of participating in video-reflexive ethnography are considerable.[25] Those who have used video footage of *in situ* activity for reflexive purposes also know that video footage portrays much more than an emaciated here and now, and that it offers much more than a paper-thin slice of organisational reality. Indeed, instead of reducing the richness of organisa-tional practices and of people's responses, video footage adds *hologrammatic* and *affective* depth.

Video's *hologrammatic* depth is evident in three ways. First, footage implicates and invokes a relevant past by reaching back in time from what is unfolding on the screen. For instance, practitioners can 'see' the resource decision that was handed down several months before the footage was shot. Second, they may be reminded of what happened following on from what is portrayed on the screen. Third, the portrayal may be extended out by the viewer to link to relevant concur-rent events they know about, related routines, and people in neighbouring spaces. In short, witnessing their activities on-screen can act as a springboard for seeing through and across the organisation of work, into the past, into the future, and out into the present organisation as a field of practices.

Video's *affective* depth is evident from what people do in response to viewing

---

25 As this book goes to press, the NICU at Maastricht Medical Centre has decided to set in train (as of December 2012) a practitioner-driven video-reflexive ethnography program to enhance their professional training and practice improvement.

themselves. This perhaps brings us the most adventurous claim in this book: exnovation using video-reflexive ethnography enables *practitioners to become open to sharing a unique and distributed intelligence*. Viewing video footage alerts people to the prevalence and pervasiveness of taken-as-given habits. Making this realisation explicit gives access to that space of habituation. At the same time, such deliberation builds people's shared (albeit distributed) intelligence.

The third objection raised above – we might film an incident that can be subpoenaed by a plaintiff lawyer – was dealt with adequately there and we will not rehearse those arguments here. Above, we concluded that if something goes wrong in health care we would expect those involved to *want* to know as much as possible about how it happened, and that they would welcome footage of things going wrong. As professionals, clinicians are bound by their professional Codes of Conduct to learn from incidents and to prevent them from happening again. On the evidence presented in this book, video footage would make it possible to enhance and enrich this process of learning.

From collective competence to distributed intelligence

People acting together tend to manifest a degree of collective competence. Their activities are likely to intersect and complement one another in ways that too often remain tacit, unarticulated. The ability to act together in this way manifests a degree of collective competence. By contrast, the ability to develop a reflexive discourse or a meta-discourse may mark the beginnings of the group intervening in its own habits and routines. Such collective intervention, particularly when it shifts from offline (away from the work) to online (at work), marks the shift from collective competence into distributed intelligence.[26]

As explained in Chapter 4, intelligence is not so much a personal as a social or 'distributed' attribute. We have attempted to corral this idea of distributed

---

26 Fisher and Ferlie distinguish ethics-oriented from rule-oriented attitudes towards dealing with clinical risk (Fisher and Ferlie, in press). Their distinction differentiates frontline practitioners initiating practice improvement 'bottom-up' from the process of 'experts elsewhere', imposing rules for action on those (practitioners) who are expected to realise those rules (guidelines, protocols, etc). Collective competence, because it is rooted in tacit habituations, may not correspond to the dictates of formal rules or guidelines, but it is slave to stable cultural rules which practitioners appropriate more or less unquestioningly. Distributed intelligence is ethics based because it involves practitioners in thinking and talking openly and critically about the effectiveness and appropriateness of their practices.

intelligence using phrases such as 'passivity competence', 'collective mindfulness', and 'weave of commitments'. Passivity competence, we learned from Sloterdijk (2009), refers to people's capacity for openness and observation, for working with uncertainty and complexity, and deferring known answers and solutions. Mindfulness refers to our awareness of and interest in what others do (Weick, 2004). Weave of commitments refers to the quality and density of our communication and relationships (Degeling, 2000). Put together, if viewing video footage induces an interest in observing *in situ* practice (passivity competence), it may alert people to the need for more attention to how they act together (mindfulness), and this may strengthen the weave of their relationships. Collectively, the outcome is enhanced intelligence, not because individuals have more knowledge, but because how they enact the processes of knowing together are better geared to handling complexity (Boreham, 2004; Manidis, 2012). In knowing with, for and alongside one another, people are better equipped to engage with complexity and produce desirable outcomes from it.

In focusing on local teams' and groups' distributed intelligence, this book has not paid much attention to large-scale system reform. Large-scale reform is often regarded as a precondition for rendering feasible, meaningful and sustainable anything that front-line practitioners may chose to undertake (Benn *et al.*, 2009). We do not deny the critical importance of structural (organisational) and super-structural (health departmental and policy) reform. These contexts of practice are often so influential as to be defining of what happens at the front line. They play a critical role in supporting front-line practice improvement initiatives and inspiring front-line excellence.

That said, we should not assume that there is a linear and logical relationship between organisational (super)structure and managerial context on the one hand, and front-line practice and individuals' activities on the other hand. To posit such a relationship risks implying that 'real' change can only occur if and when it encompasses the entire organisation and its whole hierarchy. It may also mean that we believe that (super)structural conditions predict and define front line, *in situ* practice and its potential for improvement.

We know that neither of these need be the case. The latter assumption is undermined by studies that reveal the non-compliant and 'normal–illegal' dimensions of practice (Mangione-Smith *et al.*, 2007; McGlynn *et al.*, 2003). This shows that *in situ* practice is not beholden to superstructural fiat. The former assumption comes up against studies that describe the power and achievements of local initiatives, defeating all sorts of cultural and structural constraints (Bosk *et al.*, 2009). Here, we realise that we should '[n]ever doubt that a small group of thoughtful, committed citizens can change the world. Indeed, it is the only thing that ever has.'[27]

This book has placed confidence in the ability of front-line practitioners to intervene in their own care processes and conducts, and potentially also their contexts of practice. It further advocates these people's centrality to improvement, thereby highlighting their obligation to develop shared intelligence. Such intelligence is not principally about individual people's emotional control and perspicacity (Goleman, 1995). Rather, it is about how people's relationships and communication may give a junior clinician the feeling they will be able to learn without feeling stressed about the consequences of making an error, and they may give a patient confidence that they will be looked after well.

This intelligence, then, is a social, distributed intelligence (Goleman, 2006). It is an intelligence that manifests in how practitioners perform in their moment-to-moment interactions. More so than a cognitive or emotional characteristic, this intelligence is an *affect*. Affect embodies what people do and what they *can* do together, in and through their relations (Deleuze, 2005). We suggest that affect is critical to safety (Iedema *et al.*, 2009a).

Affect has thus far not been recognised as having any importance in health care provision and quality and safety debates. The conventional view is that people's relations are 'merely' local, personal and subjective. Such a view makes *in situ* relations arbitrary to the clinical-technical matters that make up clinicians' practices and their outcomes. However, recently, patient-centred care groups and initiatives have begun to promote attention to how clinicians enact relationships with patients (Stone, 2008). Neuroscientists have begun to show, too, that relationships impact on care outcomes (Benedetti, 2011; Benedetti and Amanzio, 2011). Other scholars note that clinicians who fail to pay attention to patients' preferences commit 'silent misdiagnosis': diagnosis that reinforces the clinicians' own preconceptions at the expense of patients' far more conservative and resource-conserving preferences (Mulley *et al.*, 2012). Here, playing a critical role are respect, shared decision-making, consumer participation, and so forth (Australian Commission on Safety and Quality in Health Care, 2010). In fact, interpersonal relations and what their qualities enable people to do – the totality

---

27 This quote has been attributed to the American anthropologist Margaret Mead but it has never been located in any of her writings. It has been suggested that she may have mentioned these words to a news reporter, and that they capture an idea she presents in her book *Continuities in Cultural Evolution* (1964). In true American style, the quote has been trademarked by Sevanne Kassarjian, New York.

of *affects* – are essential to the development, sharing and growth of professional expertise and therefore to health care safety (Iedema *et al.*, 2009a).

To sum up the discussion, we suggest that viewing footage of our own work means we come to appreciate:

- the *co-constructed* nature of interaction and work: statements and actions are not the property of a specific person or specific persons but are prefigured as it were by the situation in which they find themselves;
- the *constantly changing and dynamic nature* of the 'here and now', or its constant becoming and therefore its relative openness (to change, to being different) and its open-endedness;
- the *contingent aspect of (one's own and others') self and actions*: who we are and what we do depends on and varies according to whom we are with and where we are;
- this highlights the *deep connectedness* that follows, defines and precedes us as actors and our actions.

In sum, and at the risk of closing on a truism, relationships, and not just knowledge, are critical to ensuring good outcomes in health care. What this implies is, for example, that it is not possible for clinicians lacking familiarity with patients and their complaints to properly administer treatments to those patients (Mulley *et al.*, 2012). On the same principle, it is difficult for professionals to learn their 'trade' in the absence of meaningful and intelligent relationships with those in more senior positions (Iedema *et al.*, 2009a). Of course, important knowledge may be acquired and negotiated 'objectively', as I can read a treatment guideline, a care pathway or a medication administration protocol. But knowing-*that* exists at one or more removes from *in situ* practice. Knowing-*how* – phronesis – needs to complement knowing-*that*. Knowing-how involves doing, but doing without understanding actors' reasonings, trade-offs, workarounds and shortcuts does not engender phronesis.

At this point, let us ask the following question: what exactly is the price of our conventional privileging of knowing-that (formal evidence) at the expense of knowing-how (phronesis)? Could it be that the marginalisation of phronesis, and attendant inattention to what we do and say in the here and now, are behind organisations' 'drift into failure'?

Can humans avoid drifting into failure?

Drift into failure occurs when actions become routine, and when routine allows incremental steps towards cutting corners and naturalising workarounds, as this produces conditions that are ripe for failure (Dekker, 2011). Dekker's view of humans' ability to prevent such drift is dystopian – he offers but limited hope. Going against established incident and accident investigation approaches that aim to seek out a cause or causes and eliminate them (as in 'root cause analysis'), Dekker categorically rejects the notion that there is a point to finding broken components or blameworthy decisions and actions. For him, as for us, to focus on what is broken misses all that which succeeds. To focus on what is broken is deficit thinking. It positions the practitioner as failure, it assumes that learning can only emerge from failure, and it regards failure to harbour all the learnings we may ever need to practise well and safely (Hollnagel, 2006).

Authorities, industries and services delve tirelessly into the past when investigating errors and failures. Their expectation is that the past will offer up clear causes, like broken machine components, that can be fixed or replaced. The fixing or replacement acts as an important sign. This sign says, the failure or error has been taken seriously, and our activity is a guarantor for the error or failure not happening again.

Raising questions about this approach, the stories told by people who witnessed the unfolding of such incidents generally reveal much complexity and residual uncertainty (Vaughan, 1999). But investigation reports rarely if ever make mention of such residual uncertainties. Conventional investigations target what can be known about the incident, and everything else is ignored. We look for causes (our 'keys') in places where there is light, and everything and everywhere else becomes inconsequential.

Conventional ways of addressing incidents suffer from another drawback. They betray the adherence of authorities, industries and services to what Dekker refers to as their *Cartesian-Newtonian assumptions*: reality can be controlled, causes can be isolated, aspects of how the world works can be fixed, and the system will be perfect again. These assumptions are Cartesian because they posit that we can step outside of the world, and apprehend it through 'the view from nowhere'. Such a view makes it possible to capture all the relevant causes behind what went wrong. These assumptions are Newtonian in that they regard causes as directly commensurate to their effects: what we put in is what comes out. The world and everything in it is like a machine that relays forces through isolatable and fixable components in the directions and with the intensity originally given to them. This is a world that has not yet entered the era of complexity.

The Cartesian-Newtonian world view that informs such thinking is inadequate for dealing with systems in the contemporary world. This is because the contemporary world is complex: small phenomena can cause enormous, disproportionate perturbations. Likewise, enormous investments may have limited or no effect. Our actions, as Dekker explains, 'control nothing but influence everything'. Identifying causes therefore is a way of imposing a construal of what happened on a past. However, the past's complexity is likely to defy simplistic narratives about the origin and pathway of an incident or accident. In this day and age, given practices and people in it are so interconnected and activities are so overdetermined, a single person's action is unlikely to be the sole cause of an incident. A singe person's action constitutes just a single node in a dense web of actions mediating it, contextualising it, reconfiguring it, and translating it. This web of connectedness, as we have noted, becomes evident when practice is viewed on the video screen where commonalities and continuities come to the fore.

Because of this, to understand errors and failures as issuing from specific actions or origins misses the point. Actions are themselves entangled with other actions, technologies, reactions, spaces, and so forth. Drift towards failure becomes possible (if not in fact normal; *see* Perrow's *Normal Accidents* (1984)) because actors cannot see where the totality of their activity is headed or what risks it creates and faces. This leads Dekker to claim that the system of activity is too expansive to apprehend for the individuals in it. He refers to this as the 'locality principle'. Actors are caught within the locality principle, rendering them incapable of looking at their situations and processes from the outside, with an objective eye. If anything, says Dekker, the harder and longer you look at a failure or a problem the less certain you become of how and where to place its origin, and the more you realise accidents and incidents spring from otherwise 'ordinary' ways of working, without clear locatable cause or origin.

Are we then inevitably oblivious to the threat of 'drift into failure' and are we condemned to facing 'normal accidents'? While for much of his book *Drift into Failure* this seems to be what he is saying, Dekker does offer some strategies in the very last chapter (Dekker, 2011). One set of strategies he proposes that may help tame the seemingly inevitable drift into failure and prevent normal accidents centres on what people speak about and how they speak: speaking the language of complexity – terms such as 'running to failure' may alert people to risks (p. 171); asking people to articulate how they understand the system to work (p. 180), including 'critical reflection on practice' (pp. 180, 181) and 'authentic stories'

(p. 199) and 'multiple stories' (p. 185); discussing 'unruly technology' (p. 180); finding people that say 'no' (p. 178); have different people express views and experiences (p. 173); and introducing 'fresh perspectives' (p. 186).

These strategies are complemented with the following, which centre on bringing different people together. Dekker sets store by creating diversity (p. 173), bringing in people 'from elsewhere' (p. 180), and making use of 'job rotation' (p. 180). Management can support these strategies as follows: decentralising decision-making (p. 173); managing not by directive but by 'co- and counter-evolving complexity' (p. 185), and 'taking small steps', which targets small achievements rather than system-wide ones (p. 187).

While specific, Dekker's strategies nevertheless lack clarification and exemplification. This lack denies us insight into how these strategies may be brought about, and how they may practically overcome the confounding influence of the 'locality principle' (p. 185). If actors cannot see the whole of the system, and their perspectives are therefore restricted, what might multiplying such partial perspectives produce? Can locality blindness or prejudice be defeated by deploying the strategies Dekker sets out? What guarantees that the local perspectives of actors will be expanded through telling and hearing authentic stories, encountering diversity, and so forth? Somewhat more academically, what is Dekker's view of how people *learn* to become smarter about complexity? What is his *pedagogy*?

By not articulating a clear pedagogic philosophy explaining how people can escape from or at least defer the locality principle, Dekker leaves us with the impression that systems are hellishly complex to steer, improve and direct away from failure. The efficacy of the strategies suggested here is also not self-evident, because actors' attempts at controlling systems are said to have but limited effect. This of course drastically obscures the assumed pedagogic trajectory that will lead actors from locality blindness into complexity intelligence. Not specifying this trajectory also means that other critical dimensions of learning are not clarified: how to overcome cultural habituation, how to defeat organisational politics, and how to transform professional identity.

Patient safety pedagogy

A considerable body of work has addressed the opportunities and challenges of educating people about the inertia issuing from culture, politics and hierarchy (e.g. Gherardi, 2007). One prominent early contribution in this area is John Dewey (Dewey, 1922), whose pragmatist educational philosophy has inspired a whole tradition of practice-based theories of learning (e.g. Boud and Miller, 1996). Habituation, as Dewey pointed out nearly a hundred years ago, works though the body (Dewey, 1922). Humans are predisposed to acting in ways that are legitimated, naturalised and rewarded by their culture. Issuing from and anchored in culture, habits are as easily changed as we can whistle for wind, to paraphrase Dewey. His point was that we cannot change our habits at will. Something more incisive is needed that impacts on habit: a technique through which difference and stories are given credence enough for them to begin to awaken a need for practitioners and patients to talk and nurture a shared intelligence (Iedema, 2011).

In Dewey's writings, knowings, sayings and beings are contingent on and manifested through habituated doings. The focus of educational attention, therefore, for outside analysts and for educators and employee-learners themselves, is on the embodied habits and non-human resources that structure and legitimate practice (Schatzki, 2005). Practice-based approaches to training and improvement assist practitioners with confronting how they work in the here and now. They calibrate practitioners' involvement in learning and change, acknowledging varying, contrasting and at times *conflicting* cultural and political stakes in what is status quo and what is seen to be in need of change. Such pedagogy further offers strategies not just for enabling practitioners to reconfigure the partial and partisan dimensions of their habits, knowledges and routines (Iedema and Carroll, 2011). This pedagogy also relies on concepts drawn from complexity theory about how practice change takes hold and spreads through groups and institutions, capturing, affecting or 'infecting' others.

For patients, complexity is likely to be part of their everyday experience (Cleary, 2003). What is important for them is that individual clinicians are both skilful and attentive, regardless of the competing demands placed on them. Patients are forgiving with regard to instances of inadequate technical performance, or when action confronts unavoidable problems (Iedema *et al.*, 2011). They are not forgiving, however, when they are denied respectful and attentive conduct. These points are central, and no number of up-to-the-minute technologies, time-honoured routines or well-designed systems can act as guarantor for good care. Nor can well-established habits and conventions act as excuses for bad care (Toft and Gooderham, 2009). Ignoring patients has now been identified as an important resource expenditure problem (Mulley *et al.*, 2012) and as a clear safety risk (Iedema *et al.*, 2011). With this, affect can no longer be relegated to the backbench as unimportant and inconsequential.

Where skilful practice is a technical attribute, attentiveness is an interpersonal and affect-based attribute. As such, it is a *team* attribute. Indeed, attentiveness can be seen to be a locally shared or *distributed* intelligence. Such distributed intelligence straddles people and the way they mobilise resources and spaces (Gherardi, 2007).

Having elicited it using video footage of *in situ* work practices, we have seen practitioners collaboratively produce such distributed intelligence through scrutinising their own work and strengthening their weave of mutual commitment through meta-discursive talk. The preceding case studies have indicated that such intelligence may inspire sufficient momentum to occasion learning, and thus leave locality blindness and partisan politics in its wake.

Conclusion

Exnovation builds distributed intelligence. The term 'distributed intelligence' emphasises that clinicians may experience a mutually expansive capacity, ability and confidence to act not just prospectively (planning) and retrospectively (analysis) but also creatively on and in the here and now. Strengthening the willingness and ability of clinicians to act in and on the here and now involves engendering in them *in situ* reflexivity. This, in turn, is contingent on calibrated, facilitated and repeated scrutiny of their own practices, assumptions and outcomes. This scrutiny is assisted, ideally, not just with abstract (statistical) data but also with visual and narrative data capturing the learner's own enmeshment in existing practices (Iedema, 2011; Iedema *et al.*, 2006; Kaiser Permanente, 2010).

The 'video-reflexive' approach presented in this book set out to combine a method ('video and study footage of own practice'), a rationale ('learning is conditional on embodied reflexivity') and a pedagogy ('learning arises from the interruption of taken-as-given practices and behaviours because it engenders reflexivity'). Video-reflexivity confronts clinicians with the apparently mundane and everyday dimensions of their own work. These include cultural, political, clinical, technical, personal and communicative dimensions.

The power of this approach is that visual data act as a hologram, revealing local specificities, dynamic complexities and pervasive interconnectedness. Instead of drowning in idiosyncratic specificity, subjectivity and localisms, studying one's own local practices enables clinicians to strengthen their professional capability to make more sophisticated judgements in their own and other settings and circumstances. Video-reflexive ethnography thereby embeds a pragmatic pedagogic philosophy with a practitioner-driven and outcomes-based change strategy.

Visualising health care practice improvement

In view of the rising complexity of contemporary care, practitioners' centrality to limiting that complexity, and the critical role of learning in containing that complexity, it would seem that video reflexivity can only rise in significance and broaden in its application.

Bibliography

Agar M. *The Professional Stranger: an informal introduction to ethnography*. New York, NY: Academic Press; 1980.

Alvarez G, Coiera E. Interruptive communication patterns in the intensive care unit ward round. *Int J Med Inform*. 2005; **74**(10): 791–6.

Amalberti R, Auroy Y, Berwick D, *et al*. Five system barriers to achieving ultrasafe health care. *Ann Intern Med*. 2005; **142**(9): 756–64.

Anspach R, Mizrachi N. The field worker's field: ethics, ethnography and medical sociology. *Sociol Health Illn*. 2006; **28**(6): 713–31.

Arora V, Johnson J, Lovinger D, *et al*. Communication failures in patient sign-out and suggestions for improvement: a critical incident analysis. *Qual Saf Health Care*. 2005; **14**(6): 401–7.

Australian Commission on Safety and Quality in Health Care. *The OSSIE Guide to Clinical Handover Improvement*. Sydney: Australian Commission on Safety and Quality in Health Care; 2009.

Australian Commission on Safety and Quality in Health Care. *Patient-centred Care: improving quality and safety by focusing care on patients and consumers* [discussion paper]. Sydney: Australian Commission on Safety and Quality in Health Care; 2010.

Babich BE, Bergoffen DB, Glynn SV, editors. *Continental and Postmodern Perspectives in the Philosophy of Science*. Aldershot: Avebury; 1995.

Barad K. Getting real: technoscientific practices and the materialization of reality. *Differences*. 1998; **10**(2): 87–128.

Barad K. Posthumanist performativity: toward an understanding of how matter comes to matter. *Signs*. 2003; **28**(3): 801–31.

Bate P. Changing the culture of a hospital: from hierarchy to network community. *Pub Admin Rev*. 2000; 78: 485–512.

Bate P, Robert G. Knowledge management and communities of practice in the private sector: lessons for leading the quality revolution in health care. In: Dopson S, Mark AL, editors. *Leading Health Care Organizations*. Basingstoke/New York, NY: Palgrave Macmillan; 2003. pp. 81–99.

Bate P, Robert G. *Bringing User Experience to Healthcare Improvement: the concepts, methods and practices of experience-based design*. Oxford/Seattle: Radcliffe; 2007.

Beckett S. *L'innommable* [*The Unnamable*]. Paris: Editions de Minuit; 1953.

Bibliography

Begun J, Kaissi A. Uncertainty in health care environments: myth or reality? *Health Care Manage Rev.* 2004; **29**(1): 31–9.

Benedetti F. *The Patient's Brain.* Oxford: Oxford University Press; 2011.

Benedetti F, Amanzio M. The placebo response: how words and rituals change the patient's brain. *Patient Educ Couns.* 2011; **84**(3): 413–19.

Benn J, Burnett S, Parand A, *et al.* Studying large-scale programmes to improve patient safety in whole care systems: challenges for research. *Soc Sci Med.* 2009; **69**(12): 1767–76.

Benner P. The role of articulation in understanding practice and experience as sources of knowledge in clinical nursing. In: Tully J, editor. *Philosophy in an Age of Pluralism: the philosophy of Charles Taylor in question.* Cambridge: Cambridge University Press; 1994. pp. 136–55.

Berg M. *Rationalizing Medical Work: decision-support techniques and medical practices.* Cambridge, MA: MIT Press; 1997.

Berg M. Order(s) and disorder(s): of protocols and medical practices. In: Berg M, Mol A, editors. *Differences in Medicine: unraveling practices, techniques, and bodies.* Durham/London: Duke University Press; 1998. pp. 226–46.

Berg M, Hostman K, Plass S, *et al.* Guidelines, professionals and the production of objectivity: standardization and the professionalism of insurance medicine. *Sociol Health Illn.* 2000; **22**(6): 765–91.

Berg M, Mol A. *Differences in Medicine: unraveling practices, techniques and bodies.* Durham/London: Duke University Press; 1998.

Bergs EA, Rutten FL, Tadros T, *et al.* Communication during trauma resuscitation: do we know what is happening? *Injury.* 2005; **36**(8): 905–11.

Bernstein B. *Class, Codes and Control Vol 3: Towards a Theory of Educational Transmissions.* London: Routledge & Kegan Paul; 1975.

Berwick D. A primer on leading the improvement of systems. *BMJ.* 1996; **312**(7031): 619–22.

Berwick D. *What is Evidence?* [Keynote presentation] 19th Annual National Forum on Quality Improvement in Health Care. San Francisco, California; 9–12 December 2007.

Berwick D. The science of improvement. *JAMA.* 2008; **299**(10): 1182–4.

Berwick D. What 'patient-centred' should mean: confessions of an extremist. *Health Aff (Millwood).* 2009; **28**(4): 555–65.

Bleakley A. Broadening conceptions of learning in medical education: the message from teamworking. *Med Educ.* 2006: **40**(2): 150–7.

Bliss M. *The Making of Modern Medicine: turning points in the treatment of disease.* Chicago, IL: Chicago University Press; 2011.

Bloom SW. The medical school as a social organization: the sources of resistance to change. *Med Educ.* 1989; **23**(3): 228–41.

Boreham N. A theory of collective competence: challenging the neo-liberal individualisation of performance at work. *Br J Educ Stud.* 2004; **52**(2): 5–17.

Boreham NC, Shea CE, Mackway-Jones K. Clinical risk and collective competence in the hospital emergency department in the UK. *Soc Sci Med.* 2000; **51**(1): 83–91.

Bosk CL, Dixon-Woods M, Goeschel C, *et al*. The art of medicine: reality check for checklists. *Lancet*. 2009; **374**(9688): 444–5.

Bottorff JL. Using videotaped recordings in qualitative research. In: Morse JM, editor. *Critical Issues in Qualitative Research Methods*. Thousand Oaks, CA: Sage; 1994. pp. 244–61.

Boud D, Miller N. *Working with Experience: animating learning*. London: Routledge; 1996.

Bourdieu P. *The Logic of Practice*. Cambridge: Polity Press; 1990.

Bowker G, Star SL. *Sorting Things Out*. Cambridge, MA: MIT Press; 1999.

Broekhuis M, Veldkamp C. The usefulness and feasibility of a reflexivity method to improve clinical handover. *J Eval Clin Pract*. 2007; **13**(1): 109–15.

Burke K. *A Grammar of Motives*. Englewood Cliffs, NJ: Prentice-Hall; 1969.

Campbell H, Hotchkiss R, Bradshaw N, *et al*. Integrated care pathways. *BMJ*. 1998; **316**(7125): 133–7.

Carroll JS, Edmondson AC. Leading organisational learning in health care. *Qual Saf Health Care*. 2002; **11**(1): 51–6.

Carroll K. Unpredictable predictables: complexity theory and the construction of order in intensive care [unpublished PhD thesis]. Sydney: Centre for Health Communication, University of Technology, Sydney; 2009.

Carroll K, Iedema R, Kerridge R. Reshaping ICU ward round practices using video reflexive ethnography. *Qual Health Res*. 2008; **18**(3): 380–90.

Carroll K, Mesman J. Ethnographic context meets ethnographic biography: a challenge for the mores of doing fieldwork. *Int J Mult Res Approaches*. 2012; **5**(2): 155–68.

Cleary PD. A hospitalisation from hell: a patient's perspective on quality. *Ann Int Med*. 2003; **138**(1): 33–9.

Cohen M, Hilligoss B. *Handoffs in Hospitals: a review of the literature on information exchange while transferring patient responsibility or control*. Ann Arbor: University of Michigan; 2009.

Cohen M, Hilligoss B. The published literature on handoffs in hospitals: deficiencies identified in an extensive review. *Qual Saf Health Care*. 2010; **19**(6): 493–7.

Cohen SG, Bailey DR. What makes teams work: group effectiveness research from the shop floor to the executive suite. *J Manage*. 1997; **23**(4): 238–90.

Coiera E, Jayasuriya RA, Hardy J, *et al*. Communication loads on clinical staff in the emergency department. *Med J Aust*. 2002; **176**(9): 415–18.

Coiera E, Tombs V. Communication behaviours in a hospital setting: an observational study. *BMJ*. 1998; **316**(7132): 673–6.

Cooperrider DL, Whitney D. *Appreciative Enquiry*. San Francisco, CA: Berret-Koehler; 1999.

Damasio A. *Descartes' Error: emotion, reason and the human brain*. London/New York, NY: Penguin; 1994.

Damasio A. *Looking for Spinoza: joy, sorrow and the feeling brain*. London: Vintage; 2003.

De Wilde R. *Innovating Innovation: a contribution to the philosophy of the future*. Paper read at the Policy Agendas for Sustainable Technological Innovation Conference, London; 1–3 December, 2000.

Bibliography

Deacon T. *The Symbolic Species: the co-evolution of language and brain*. Harmondsworth: Penguin; 1997.

Deetz S. *Transforming Communication, Transforming Business: building responsive and responsible workplaces*. Cresskill, NJ: Hampton Press; 1995.

Degeling P. Reconsidering clinical accountability: an examination of some dilemmas inherent in efforts to bolster clinician accountability. *Int J Health Plann Manage*. 2000; **15**(1): 3–16.

Degeling P, Sorensen R, Maxwell S, *et al. The Organisation of Hospital Care and its Effects*. Sydney: Centre for Hospital Management and Information Systems Research, The University of New South Wales; 2001.

Dekker S. *Ten Questions about Human Error: a new view of human factors and system safety*. Mahwah, NJ: Lawrence Erlbaum; 2005.

Dekker S. *Just Culture*. Aldershot: Ashgate; 2008.

Dekker S. *Drift into Failure*. Aldershot: Ashgate; 2011.

Deleuze G. Ethology: Spinoza and us. In: Fraser M, Greco M, editors. *The Body: a reader*. London: Routledge; 2005. pp. 58–61.

Dewey J. *Democracy and Education*. New York: The Macmillan Company; 1944.

Dewey J. *Human Nature and Conduct: an introduction to social psychology*. New York, NY: H Holt; 1922.

Dewey J. *Reconstruction in Philosophy*. New York, NY: Courier Dover; 2004.

Dreyfus H. *What Computers Can't Do*. New York, NY: Harper & Row; 1979.

Duhigg C. *The Power of Habits: why we do what we do in life and business*. New York, NY: Random House; 2012.

Eco U. *Semiotics and the Philosophy of Language*. London: Macmillan Press; 1984.

Edelman G. *Bright Air, Brilliant Fire: on the matter of the mind*. Harmondsworth: Penguin; 1992.

Endsley MR. Situation awareness: progress and directions. In: Banbury S, Tremblay S, editors. *A Cognitive Approach to Situation Awareness: theory, measurement and application*. Aldershot: Ashgate; 2004. pp. 317–41.

Engeström Y. *From Teams to Knots: activity-theoretical studies of collaboration and learning at work*. Cambridge/New York, NY: Cambridge University Press; 2008.

Eraut M. Informal learning in the workplace. *Stud Cont Educ*. 2004; **26**(2): 247–73.

Espin S, Lingard L, Baker GR, *et al.* Persistence of unsafe practice in everyday work: an exploration of organizational and psychological factors constraining safety in the operating room. *Qual Saf Health Care*. 2006; **15**(3): 165–70.

Evans D. *Values in Medicine: what are we really doing to patients?* London: Routledge-Cavendish; 2008.

Evans SM, Murray A, Patrick I, *et al.* Clinical handover in the trauma setting: a qualitative study of paramedics and trauma team members. *Qual Saf Health Care*. 2010; **19**(6): e57. Epub 2010 Aug 10.

Feyerabend P. *Against Method: outline of an anarchistic theory of knowledge*. New York, NY: Humanities Press; 1975.

Finn R. The language of teamwork: reproducing professional divisions in the operating theatre. *Hum Relat*. 2008; **61**(1): 103–30.

Fisher M, Ferlie EB. Resisting Hybridisation between Modes of Clinical Risk Management: Contradiction, Contest, and the Production of Intractable Conflict. *Account Org & Soc*. In Press.

Flyvbjerg B. *Making Social Science Matter: why social science fails and how it can succeed again*. Cambridge: Cambridge University Press; 2001.

Forsyth R. Tricky technology, troubled tribes: a video ethnographic study of the impact of information technology on health care professionals' practices and relationships [unpublished PhD thesis]. Sydney: School of Public Health and Community Medicine, The University of NSW; 2006.

Foucault M. *The Birth of the Clinic: an archeology of medical perception*. New York, NY: Vintage; 1973.

Garfinkel H. 'Good' organizational reasons for 'bad' clinic records. In: Garfinkel H. *Studies in Ethnomethodology*. Englewood Cliffs, NJ: Prentice Hall; 1967. pp. 186–207.

Garfinkel H. Studies of the routine grounds of everyday activities. In: Sudnow D, editor. *Studies in Social Interaction*. New York, NY: The Free Press; 1972. pp. 1–30.

Gasser L. The integration of computing and routine work. *ACM T Off Inf Syst*. 1986; **4**(3): 205–25.

Gherardi S. *Organizational Knowledge: the texture of workplace learning*. Oxford: Blackwell; 2007.

Gherardi S, Nicolini D. Learning the trade: a culture of safety in practice. *Organization*. 2002; **9**(2): 191–223.

Glaser B, Strauss A. *Awareness of Dying*. London: Weidenfeld & Nicholson; 1965.

Glaser B, Strauss A. *Time for Dying*. Chicago, IL: Aldine; 1968.

Goleman D. *Emotional Intelligence*. New York, NY: Bantham; 1995.

Goleman D. *Social Intelligence: the new science of human relationships*. London: Hutchinson; 2006.

Greatbatch D, Murphy E, Dingwall R. Evaluating medical information systems: ethnomethodological and interactionist approaches. *Health Serv Manage Res*. 2011; **14**(3): 181–91.

Greenhalgh T, Russell J, Ashcroft RE, *et al*. Why national e-health programs need dead philosophers: Wittgensteinian reflections on policymakers' reluctance to learn from history. *Millbank Q*. 2011; **89**(4): 533–63.

Greenhalgh T, Russell J, Swinglehurst D. Narrative methods in quality improvement research. *Qual Saf Health Care*. 2005; **14**(6): 443–9.

Grol R, Berwick DM, Wensing M. On the trail of quality and safety in health care. *BMJ*. 2008; **336**(7635): 74–6.

Haig KM, Sutton S, Whittington J. SBAR: a shared mental model for improving communication between clinicians. *Jt Comm J Qual Patient Saf*. 2006; **32**(3): 167–75.

Hardt M. Foreword: what affects are good for. In: Ticineto-Clough P, Halley J, editors. *The affective turn: theorizing the social*. Durham: Duke University Press; 2007. pp. ix–xiii.

Hargie OD, Morrow NC. Using videotape in communication skills training: a critical evaluation of the process of self-viewing. *Med Teach*. 1986; **8**(4): 359–65.

Bibliography

Harré R. *The Philosophies of Science: an introductory survey*. Oxford: Oxford University Press; 1972.

Harrison S, Moran M, Wood B. Policy emergence and policy convergence: the case of 'scientific-bureaucratic medicine' in the United States and United Kingdom. *Br J Polit Int Rel*. 2002; **4**(1): 1–24.

Hart MK, Hart RF. *Statistical Process Control for Health Care*. Pacific Grove, CA: Duxbury; 2002.

Heath C, Hindmarsh J. Analysing interaction: video, ethnography and situated conduct. In: May T, editor. *Qualitative Research in Action*. London: Sage; 2002. pp. 99–112.

Hitchcock CH, Dowrick PW, Prater M. Video self-modeling intervention in school-based settings: a review. *Rem Spec Educ*. 2003; **24**: 36–45.

Hollnagel E. Resilience: the challenge of the unstable. In: Hollnagel E, Woods DD, Leveson N, editors. *Resilience Engineering: concepts and precepts*. Aldershot: Ashgate; 2006. pp. 9–18.

Hollnagel E. Resilient health care: from safety I to safety II. Workshop presentation, *BMJ Patient Safety Forum*. Paris; 17–20 April, 2012.

Hollnagel E, Woods DD, Leveson N. *Resilience Engineering: concepts and precepts*. Aldershot: Ashgate; 2006.

Horn SD, Gassaway J. Practice-based evidence study design for comparative effectiveness research. *Med Care*. 2007; **45**(10 Suppl.): S50–7.

Hutchins E. *Cognition in the Wild*. Cambridge, MA: MIT Press; 1995.

Hutchins E, Klausen T. Distributed cognition in an airline cockpit. In: Engeström Y, Middleton D, editors. *Cognition and Communication at Work*. Cambridge: Cambridge University Press; 1998. pp. 15–34.

Iedema R. Creating safety by strengthening clinicians' capacity for reflexivity. *BMJ Qual Saf*. 2011; **20**(Suppl. 1): S83–6.

Iedema R, Allen S, Britton K, *et al*. Patients' and family members' views on how clinicians enact and how they should enact incident disclosure: the '100 patient stories' qualitative study. *BMJ*. 2011; **343**: d4423.

Iedema R, Allen S, Britton K, *et al*. What do patients and relatives know about problems and failures in care? *BMJ Qual Saf*. 2012a; **21**(3): 198–205. Epub 2011 Dec 16.

Iedema R, Ball C, Daly B, *et al*. Design and trial of a new ambulance-to-emergency department handover protocol: 'IMIST-AMBO'. *BMJ Qual Saf*. 2012b; **21**(8): 627–33. Epub 2012 May 23.

Iedema R, Braithwaite J, Sorensen R. The reification of numbers: statistics and the distance between self, work and others. *BMJ*. 2003; **326**: 771.

Iedema R, Carroll K. The 'clinalyst': institutionalizing reflexive space to realize safety and flexible systematization in health care. *J Organ Change Manag*. 2011; **24**(2): 175–90.

Iedema R, Degeling P, White L, *et al*. Analysing discourse practices in organisations. *Qual Res J*. 2004; **4**(1): 5–25.

Iedema R, Forsyth R, Georgiou A, *et al*. Video-research in health: visibilizing the effects of computerizing clinical care. *Qual Res J*. 2007; **6**(2): 15–30.

Iedema R, Jorm C, Lum M. Affect is central to patient safety: the horror stories of young anaesthetists. *Soc Sci Med*. 2009a; **69**(12): 1750–6.

Iedema R, Jorm C, Wakefield J, *et al.* Practising open disclosure: clinical incident communication and systems improvement. *Sociol Health Illn.* 2009b; **31**(2): 262–77.

Iedema R, Long D, Carroll K. Corridor communication, spatial design and patient safety: enacting and managing complexities. In: Van Marrewijk A, Yanow D, editors. *Space, Meaning and Organisation.* Cheltenham: Edward Elgar; 2010. pp. 41–57.

Iedema R, Long D, Forsyth R, *et al.* Visibilizing clinical work: video ethnography in the contemporary hospital. *Health Sociol Rev.* 2006; **15**(2): 156–68.

Iedema R, Mallock N, Sorensen R, *et al.* The National Open Disclosure Pilot: evaluation of a policy implementation initiative. *Med J Aust.* 2008; **188**(7): 397–400.

Iedema R, Merrick E. '*Handover – Enabling Learning in Communication for Safety*' *(HELICS)': a DVD/booklet-based kit for handover improvement.* Sydney: Australian Commission on Safety and Quality in Health Care; University of Technology, Sydney; 2008.

Iedema R, Merrick E. Team work in health care: how clinicians negotiate the continuity of clinical tasks and care responsibilities. In: Sarangi S, Linel, P, editors. *Team Talk: decision-making across boundaries in health and social care.* London: Equinox; 2013.

Iedema R, Merrick E, Daly B, *et al. Telling It Like It Is: people's experiences of an emergency department* [DVD]. Australia: Centre for Health Communication; 2009c.

Iedema R, Merrick E, Kerridge R, *et al.* 'Handover – Enabling Learning in Communication for Safety' (HELICS): a report on achievements at two hospital sites. *Med J Aust.* 2009d; **190**(11 Suppl.): S133–6.

Iedema R, Merrick E, Piper D, *et al.* Co-design as discursive practice in emergency health services: the architecture of deliberation. *J Appl Behav Sci.* 2010; **46**(2010): 73–91.

Iedema R, Merrick E, Rajbhandari D, *et al.* Viewing the taken-for-granted from under a different aspect: a video-based method in pursuit of patient safety. *Int J Mult Res Approaches.* 2009e; **3**(3): 290–301.

Iedema R, Rhodes C. An ethics of mutual care in organizational surveillance. *Organ Stud.* 2010; **31**: 199–217.

Illich I. *Limits to Medicine: medical nemesis, or the expropriation of health.* London: Marion Boyars; 1976.

Innes JE, Booher DE. Consensus building as role playing and bricolage: toward a collaborative theory of planning. *J Am Plann Assoc.* 1999; **65**(1): 9–25.

Jeffers JM, Guthrie DW. Self-assessment via videotaping to maximize teaching effectiveness. *J Contin Educ Nurs.* 1988; **19**(5): 223–6.

Johnson BH, Abraham MR. *Partnering with Patients, Residents and Families: a resource for leaders of hospitals, ambulatory care settings, and long-term care communities.* Bethesda, MD: Institute for Patient- and Family-Centered Care; 2012.

Jorm C. *Reconstructing Medical Practice: engagement, professionalism and critical relationships in health care.* Farnham, UK: Gower; 2012.

Jorm C, White S, Kaneen T. Clinical handover: critical communications. *Med J Aust.* 2009; **190**(11 Suppl.): S108–9.

Kahneman D, Klein G. Conditions for intuitive expertise. *Am Psychol.* 2009; **64**(6): 515–26.

Bibliography

Kaiser Permanente. *Getting Started in Video Ethnography: a catalyst for guiding and motivating quality improvement*. Oakland, CA: Kaiser Permanente Care Management Institute; 2010.

Kennedy M. Generalizing from single case studies. *Eval Rev*. 1979; **3**(4): 661–78.

Klein G. *Sources of Power: how people make decisions*. Cambridge, MA: MIT Press; 1999.

Klein G, Baxter H. *Cognitive Transformation Theory: contrasting cognitive and behavioral learning*. Interservice/Industry Training, Simulation, and Education Conference (I/ITSEC) 2006, Orlando, Florida; 1–4 May, 2006.

Kornberger M, Clegg S. Bringing space back in: organizing the generative building. *Organ Stud*. 2004; **25**(7): 1095–115.

Kuhn TS. *The Structure of Scientific Revolutions*. Chicago, IL: University of Chicago Press; 1962.

Kunda G. *Engineering Culture: control and commitment in a high-tech corporation*. Philadelphia, PA: Temple University Press; 1992.

Langewitz W. Beyond content analysis and non-verbal behaviour: what about atmosphere? A phenomenological approach. *Patient Educ Couns*. 2007; **67**(3): 319–23.

Latour B. Visualization and cognition: thinking with eyes and hands. *Knowledge and Society*. 1986; **6**: 1–40.

Latour B. Why has critique run out of steam? From matters of fact to matters of concern. *Critical Inquiry*. 2004; **30**(2): 225–48.

Latour B. *Reassembling the Social: an introduction to actor-network theory*. Oxford: Oxford University Press; 2005.

Latour B, Woolgar S. *Laboratory Life: the social construction of scientific facts*. London: Sage; 1979.

Lave J. The practice of learning. In: Chaiklin S, Lave J, editors. *Understanding Practice: perspectives on activity and context*. Cambridge: Cambridge University Press; 1993. pp. 3–32.

Lave J, Wenger E. *Situated Learning: legitimate peripheral participation*. Cambridge: Cambridge University Press; 1990.

Law J, Mol A. *Complexities: social studies of knowledge practices*. Durham, NC/London: Duke University Press; 2002.

Leape L, Berwick D, Bates D. What practices will most improve safety? Evidence-based medicine meets patient safety. *J Am Med Assoc*. 2002; **288**(4): 501–7.

Lemieux-Charles L, McGuire WL. What do we know about health care team effectiveness? A review of the literature. *Med Care Res Rev*. 2006; **63**(3): 263–300.

Lief HI, Fox, RC. Training for 'detached concern' in medical students. In: Lief HI, Lief VF, Lief NR, editors. *The Psychological Basis of Medical Practice*. New York: Harper Row; 1963. pp. 12–35.

Lillrank P, Liukko M. Standard, routine and non-routine processes in health care. *Int J Health Care Qual Assur Inc Leadersh Health Serv*. 2004; **17**(1): 39–46.

Lingard L, Espin S, Rubin B, *et al*. Getting teams to talk: development and pilot implementation of a checklist to promote interprofessional communication in the OR. *Qual Saf Health Care*. 2005; **14**(5): 340–6.

Lingard L, Reznick R, DeVito I, *et al*. Forming professional identities on the health care team: discursive constructions of the 'other' in the operating room. *Med Educ.* 2002; **36**(8): 728–34.

Little M. *Humane Medicine.* Sydney: Allen & Unwin; 1994.

Lohr K. Emerging methods in comparative effectiveness and safety: symposium overview and summary. *Med Care.* 2007; **45**(10 Suppl. 2): S5–8.

London Ambulance Service. Procedure relating to the clinical handover of patients. London: National Health Service UK; 2008.

MacDougall D. *The Corporeal Image: film, ethnography and the senses.* Princeton, NJ: Princeton University Press; 2006.

Mackenzie CF, Xiao Y. Video techniques and data compared with observation in emergency trauma care. *Qual Saf Health Care.* 2003; **12**(Suppl 2): ii51–7.

Mangione-Smith R, De Cristofaro AH, Setodji CM, *et al.* The quality of ambulatory care delivered to children in the United States. *N Engl J Med.* 2007; **357**(15): 1515–23.

Manidis M. *Practising Knowing in Emergency Departments: tracing the disciplinary, institutional and spatio-temporal complexities of working/knowing practices in modern emergency department care* [unpublished PhD thesis]. Sydney: University of Technology, Sydney; 2013.

Manidis M, Scheeres H. Towards understanding workplace learning through theorising practice: at work in hospital emergency departments. In: Hager P, Lee A, Reich A, editors. *Practice, Learning and Change: practice-theory perspectives on professional learning.* Dordrecht: Springer; 2012. pp. 103–18.

Martin JR. *Life as a Noun: arresting the universe in science and humanities.* London: Falmer Press; 1993.

Martin V. *Developing a Narrative Approach to Healthcare Research.* Oxford: Radcliffe; 2011.

Massumi B. *Parables for the Virtual: movement, affect, sensation.* Durham NC: Duke University Press; 2002.

McDonald TB, Helmchen LA, Smith KM, *et al.* Responding to patient safety incidents: the 'seven pillars'. *Qual Saf Health Care.* 2010; **19**(6); e11.

McGlynn EA, Asch SM, Adams J, *et al.* The quality of health care delivered to adults in the United States. *N Engl J Med.* 2003; **348**(26): 2635–45.

Menzies-Lyth IEP. *The Dynamics of the Social: selected essays (Volume 2).* London: Free Association Books; 1988.

Mertens DM. *Transformative Research and Evaluation.* New York, NY: Guildford Press; 2009.

Mesman J. Disturbing observations as a basis for collaborative research. *Sci Cult.* 2007; **16**(3): 281–95.

Mesman J. *Uncertainty in Medical Innovation: experienced pioneers in neonatal care.* Hampshire: Palgrave MacMillan; 2008.

Mesman J. The geography of patient safety: a topical analysis of sterility. *Soc Sci Med.* 2009; **69**(12): 705–1712.

Mesman J. Resources of strength: an exnovation of hidden competences to preserve patient safety. In: Rowley E, Waring J, editors. *A Sociocultural Perspective on Patient Safety.* Farnham, UK: Ashgate; 2011. pp. 71–92.

Bibliography

Mesman J. The relocation of vulnerability in critical care medicine. In: Hommels A, Mesman J, Bijker W, editors. *The Vulnerability of Technological Culture*. The MIT Press, forthcoming.

Mezirow J. Transformative learning: theory to practice. *New Dir Adult Cont Educ*. 1997; **1997**(74): 5–12.

Michaelson M, Levi L. Video-taping in the admitting area: a most useful tool for the quality improvement of the trauma care. *Eur J Emerg Med*. 1997; **4**(2): 94–6.

Mitchell S. *Unsimple Truths: science, complexity and policy*. Chicago, IL: Chicago University Press; 2009.

Mohr J, Batalden P, Barach P. Integrating patient safety into the clinical microsystem. *Qual Saf Health Care*. 2004; **13**(Suppl. 2): ii34–8.

Montuori A. The complexity of improvisation and the improvisation of complexity: social science, art and creativity. *Human Relations*. 2003; **56**(2): 237–55.

Mulley A, Trimble C, Elwyn G. Stop the silent misdiagnosis: patients' preferences matter. *BMJ*. 8 November 2012; **345**: e6572.

Nagel T. *The View from Nowhere*. Oxford: Oxford University Press; 1989.

Nagpal K, Arora S, Abboudi M, *et al*. Postoperative handover: problems, pitfalls, and prevention of error. *Ann Surg*. 2010; **252**(1): 171–6.

Neuwirth EB, Bellows J, Jackson AH, *et al*. How Kaiser Permanente uses video ethnography of patients for quality improvement. *Health Aff (Millwood)*. 2012; **31**(6): 1244–50.

New South Wales Health. *The NSW Health Clinical Handover Toolkit*. Sydney, Australia: New South Wales Department of Health; 2009.

Nicolini D. Practice as the site of knowing: insights from the field of telemedicine. *Organ Sci*. 2011; **22**: 602–20.

Nimnuan C, Hotopf M, Wessely S. Medically unexplained symptoms: an epidemiological study in seven specialities. *J Psychosom Res*. 2001; **51**(1): 361–7.

Norman DA. *The Psychology of Everyday Things*. New York, NY: Basic Books; 1988.

Nugus P, Carroll K, Hewett D, *et al*. Integrated care in the emergency department: a complex adaptive systems perspective. *Soc Sci Med*. 2010; **71**(11): 1997–2004.

Osler W. *The Principles and Practice of Medicine*. New York, NY: Appleton; 1892.

O'Toole M, Shukman A. A contextual glossary of formalist critical terminology. In: O'Toole M, Shukman A, editors. *Russian Poetics in Translation (Volume 4)*. Oxford: Holdan Books; 1977. pp. 1–45.

Ovretveit J. Understanding the conditions for improvement: research to discover which context influences affect improvement success. *BMJ Qual Saf*. 2011; **20**(Suppl. 1): i18–23.

Owen C, Wackers G, Béguin P. *Risky Work Environment: reappraising human work within fallible systems*. Aldershot: Ashgate; 2009.

Palmer P. A new professional: the aims of education revisited. *Change*. 2007; **39**(6): 5–12.

Park P. Knowledge and participatory research. In: Reason P, Bradbury H, editors. *Handbook of Action Research: participative enquiry and practice*. London: Sage; 1999. pp. 81–90.

Patterson ES, Cook RI, Woods D, *et al*. Gaps and resilience. In: Bogner MS, editor. *Human Error in Medicine*. Mahwah, NJ: Lawrence Erlbaum Associates; forthcoming.

Perrow C. *Normal Accidents: living with high-risk technologies*. New York, NY: Basic Books; 1984.

Pinder R, Petchey R, Shaw S, *et al*. What's in a care pathway? Towards a cultural cartography of the new NHS. *Sociol Health Illn*. 2005; **27**(6): 759–79.

Pink S. *Doing Visual Ethnography: images, media and representation in research*. London: Sage; 2001.

Pink S. *Visual Interventions*. Oxford: Berghahn; 2007.

Pope C, Mort M, Goodwin D, *et al*. Anaesthetic talk in surgical encounters. In: Iedema R, editor. *Discourses of Hospital Communication: tracing complexities in health care practices*. Basingstoke: Palgrave; 2007. pp. 161–81.

Porter R. *Enlightenment*. Basingstoke: Palgrave; 2001.

Prigogine I. *The End of Certainty: time, chaos and the new laws of nature*. New York, NY: The Free Press; 1996.

Prigogine I, Stengers I. *Order Out of Chaos: man's new dialogue with nature*. New York, NY: Bantam; 1984.

Pronovost P, Needham D, Berenholtz S, *et al*. An intervention to decrease catheter-related bloodstream infections in the ICU. *N Engl J Med*. 2006; **355**(26): 2725–32.

Quaid D, Thao J, Denham CR. Story power: the secret weapon. *J Patient Saf*. 2010; **6**(1): 5–14.

Rabøl LI, Andersen ML, Østergaard D, *et al*. Descriptions of verbal communication errors between staff: an analysis of 84 root cause analysis-reports from Danish hospitals. *BMJ Qual Saf*. 2011; **20**(3): 268–74.

Reason J. Beyond the organisational accident: the need for 'error wisdom' on the frontline. *Qual Saf Health Care*. 2004; **13**(Suppl. 2): ii28–33.

Reason P. Integrating action and reflection through co-operative inquiry. *Management Learning*. 1999; **30**(2): 207–26.

Reason P, Bradbury, H. *The Sage Handbook of Action Research: participative inquiry and practice*. London: Sage; 2008.

Richmond C, Merrick E, Green T, *et al*. Bedside review of patient care in an emergency department: the Cow Round. *Emerg Med Australas*. 2011; **23**(5): 600–5. Epub 2011 Jun 30.

Riesenberg LA, Leitzsch J, Little BW. Systematic review of handoff mnemonics literature. *Am J Med Qual*. 2009; **24**(3): 196–204.

Rossi-Landi F. *Linguistics and Economics*. The Hague: Mouton; 1975.

Rouch J. *Cine-ethnography*. Minneapolis: University of Minnesota Press; 2003.

Rowley E. Deviantly innovative: when risking patient safety is the right thing to do. In: Rowley E, Waring J, editors. *A Socio-Cultural Perspective on Patient Safety*. Farnham: Ashgate; 2011. pp. 95–113.

Runciman W, Merry A, Walton M. *Safety and Ethics in Health Care*. Aldershot: Ashgate; 2007.

Russell J, Greenhalgh T, Byrne E, *et al*. Recognizing rhetoric in health care policy analysis. *J Health Serv Res Policy*. 2008; **13**(1): 40–6.

Santora TA, Trooskin SZ, Blank CA, *et al*. Video assessment of trauma response. *Am J Emerg Med*. 1996; **14**(6): 564–9.

Bibliography

Schatzki T. The sites of organizations. *Organ Stud.* 2005; **26**: 465–84.

Schiff GD, Hasan O, Kim S, *et al*. Diagnostic error in medicine: analysis of 583 physician-reported errors. *Arch Int Med.* 2009; **169**(20): 1881–7.

Schön D. *The Reflective Practitioner: how professionals think in action.* New York, NY: Basic Books; 1983.

Schouten LM, Hulscher MEJ, Everdingen JJ, *et al*. Evidence for the impact of quality improvement collaboratives: systematic review. *BMJ.* 2008; **336**(7659): 1491–4.

Shem S. *The House of God.* London: Black Swan; 1978.

Shojania K, Duncan B, McDonald K, *et al. Making Health Care Safer: a critical analysis of patient safety practices. Evidence Report/Technology Assessment 43.* Rockville MD: Agency for Health Research and Quality; 2001.

Shojania KG, Grimshaw JM. Evidence-based quality improvement: the state of the science. *Health Aff (Millwood).* 2005; **24**(1): 138–51.

Shusterman R. *Body Consciousness: a philosophy of mindfulness and somaesthetics.* Cambridge: Cambridge University Press; 2008.

Skogstad W. Working in a world of bodies: a medical ward. In: Hinshelwood RD, Skogstad W, editors. *Observing Organisations: anxiety, defence and culture in health care.* London: Routledge; 2000. pp. 101–21.

Sloterdijk P. *Critique of Cynical Reason.* Minneapolis: University of Minnesota Press; 1984.

Sloterdijk P. *Du mußt dein Leben ändern: Über Anthropotechnik.* Frankfurt: Suhrkamp; 2009.

Smith A, Goodwin D, Mort M, *et al*. Expertise in practice: an ethnographic study exploring acquisition and use of knowledge in anaesthesia. *Br J Anaesth.* 2003; **91**(3): 319–28.

Smith AF, Pope C, Goodwin D, *et al*. Interprofessional handover and patient safety in anaesthesia: observational study of handovers in the recovery room. *Br J Anaesth.* 2008; **101**(3): 332–7.

Solet DJ, Norvell JM, Rutan GH, *et al*. Lost in translation: challenges and opportunities in physician-to-physician communication during patient handoffs. *Acad Med.* 2005; **80**(12): 1094–9.

Star SL. The politics of formal representations: wizards, gurus and organizational complexity. In: Star SL, editor. *Ecologies of Knowledge: work and politics in science and technology.* Albany: State University of New York; 1995. pp. 88–118.

Star SL, Strauss A. Layers of silence; arenas of voice: the ecology of visible and invisible work. *Computer Supported Cooperative Work.* 1999; **8**(1–2): 9–30.

Steinberg E, Luce B. Evidence based? Caveat emptor! *Health Aff (Millwood).* 2005; **24**(1): 80–93.

Stone S. A retrospective evaluation of the impact of the Planetree patient-centered model of care on inpatient quality outcomes. *HERD.* 2008; **1**(4): 55–69.

Strauss A, Schatzman L, Ehrlich D, *et al*. The hospital and its negotiated order. In: Freidson E, editor. *The Hospital in Modern Society.* New York, NY: Free Press of Glencoe; 1963. pp. 147–69.

Street RL Jr, Makoul G, Arora N, *et al*. How does communication heal? Pathways linking clinician-patient communication to health outcomes. *Patient Educ Couns.* 2009; **74**(3): 295–301.

Studdert DM, Piper D, Iedema R. Legal aspects of open disclosure II: attitudes of health professionals; findings from a national survey. *Med J Aust.* 2010; **193**(9): 351–5.

Studer Q. *Hardwiring Excellence.* Gulf Breeze, FL: Fire Starter Publishing; 2003.

Suchman L. *Plans and Situated Actions: the problem of human-machine communication.* Cambridge: Cambridge University Press; 1987.

Taylor C. *Philosophy and the Human Sciences (Philosophical Papers Volume 2).* Cambridge: Cambridge University Press; 1985.

Thakore S, Morrison W. A survey of the perceived quality of patient handover by ambulance staff in the resuscitation room. *Emerg Med J.* 2001; **18**(4): 293–6.

Thomas V. *Yumi Piksa: community-responsive filmmaking as research practice in highlands Papua New Guinea* [PhD thesis]. Sydney: Centre for Health Communication, University of Technology, Sydney; 2011.

Thrift N. *Non-representational Theory.* London: Routledge; 2008.

Ticineto-Clough P. The affective turn: political economy, biomedia and bodies. *Theor Cult Soc.* 2008; **25**(1): 1–22.

Timmermans S, Berg M. *The Gold Standard: the challenge of evidence-based medicine and standardization in health care.* Philadelphia, PA: Temple University Press; 2003.

Toft B, Gooderham P. Involuntary automaticity: a potential legal defence against an allegation of clinical negligence? *Qual Saf Health Care.* 2009; **18**(1): 69–73.

US Institute of Medicine. *To Err is Human: building a safer health system.* Washington, DC: National Academy Press; 1999.

US Joint Commission. *The Joint Commission National Patient Safety Goals.* Oakbrook Terrace, Il: US Joint Commission; 2012.

Vaughan D. The dark side of organizations: mistake, misconduct and disaster. *Ann Rev Sociol.* 1999; **25**: 271–305.

Vincent C. *Patient Safety.* London: Churchill-Livingstone/Elsevier; 2006.

Vincent CA. *Patient Safety.* 2nd ed. Oxford: Wiley-Blackwell; 2010.

Vygotsky L. *Thought and Language.* A Kozulin, trans. Cambridge, MA: MIT Press; 1986.

Wears RL, Nemeth CP. Replacing hindsight with insight: toward better understanding of diagnostic failures. *Ann Emerg Med.* 2007; **49**(2): 206–9.

Wears RL, Perry SJ, Anders S, *et al.* Resilience in the emergency department. In: Hollnagel E, Nemeth CP, Dekker SWA, editors. *Remaining Sensitive to the Possibility of Failure.* Aldershot: Ashgate; 2008. pp. 193–210.

Weick K. *Sense-Making in Organisations.* London: Sage Publications; 1995.

Weick K. Reduction of medical errors through mindful interdependence. In: Sutcliffe K, Rosenthal M, editors. *Medical Error.* San Francisco, CA: Jossey-Bass; 2004. pp. 177–99.

Weick K, Roberts KH. Collective mind in organizations: heedful interrelating on flight decks. *Admin Sci Quart.* 1993; **38**(3): 357–81.

Wittgenstein L. *Philosophical Investigations.* G Anscombe, trans. Oxford: Blackwell; 1953.

World Health Organization. *Action on Patient Safety: High 5s.* Geneva: World Health Organization; 2008.

World Health Organization; Joint Commission International. *Communication During*

Bibliography

Patient Hand-Overs. Patient safety solutions 1. Geneva: World Health Organization; 2007.

Zuiderent-Jerak T. Preventing implementation: exploring interventions with standardization in healthcare. *Sci Cult.* 2007; **16**(3): 311–29.

Zwarenstein M, Goldman J, Reeves S. Interprofessional collaboration: effects of practice-based interventions on professional practice and healthcare outcomes. Cochrane Database Syst Rev. 2009; (3): CD000072.

Index

Entries in *italics* denote figures; entries in **bold** denote tables.

Index

Index

CPD with Radcliffe

You can now use a selection of our books to achieve CPD (Continuing Professional Development) points through directed reading.

We provide a free online form and downloadable certificate for your appraisal portfolio. Look for the CPD logo and register with us at: www.radcliffehealth.com/cpd

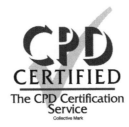